NIACIN:
The Real Story

Abram Hoffer, M.D., Ph.D.
Andrew W. Saul, Ph.D.
and Harold D. Foster, Ph.D.

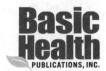

Basic Health
PUBLICATIONS, INC.

The information contained in this book is based upon the research and personal and professional experiences of the authors. It is not intended as a substitute for consulting with your physician or other healthcare provider. Any attempt to diagnose and treat an illness should be done under the direction of a healthcare professional.

The publisher does not advocate the use of any particular healthcare protocol but believes the information in this book should be available to the public. The publisher and authors are not responsible for any adverse effects or consequences resulting from the use of the suggestions, preparations, or procedures discussed in this book. Should the reader have any questions concerning the appropriateness of any procedures or preparation mentioned, the authors and the publisher strongly suggest consulting a professional healthcare advisor.

Basic Health Publications, Inc.
28812 Top of the World Drive
Laguna Beach, CA 92651
949-715-7327 • www.basichealthpub.com

Library of Congress Cataloging-in-Publication Data is available from the Library of Congress.

Editor: Karen Anspach
Interior design and production: Gary A. Rosenberg
Cover design: Mike Stromberg

Printed in the United States of America

10   9   8   7   6   5   4   3   2   1

Contents

*To all the physicians who have
demonstrated that niacin cures disease,
with particular honor to
Joseph Goldberger,
William Kaufman,
Rudolph Altschul,
Edmond Boyle,
William B. Parsons,
Humphry Osmond,
and Abram Hoffer.*

Acknowledgements

We would like to thank Steven Carter, Executive Director of the International Schizophrenia Foundation, for kind permission to use material that originally appeared in the *Journal of Orthomolecular Medicine*. I am indebted to the late Mrs. Charlotte Kaufman for gracious encouragement and permission to publish correspondence, private notes, and other writings of her husband, Dr. William Kaufman, thus making his important work widely available to the public. We value the specialized input from Dr. Robert G. Smith, Research Associate Professor in the Department of Neuroscience, University of Pennsylvania. Thanks to all the contributors to the Orthomolecular Medicine News Service, some articles of which are incorporated in this book. A special thanks to Dr. W. Todd Penberthy, for reading and making expert suggestions to the text.

Foreword

Niacin raises good cholesterol (HDL) more than any known pharmaceutical, while simultaneously lowering total cholesterol, triglycerides, and the most pathogenic form of cholesterol-associated lipoprotein (VLDL). This wide array of generally clinically desirable chemical adjustments is undeniable based on precise biochemical measures. Niacin (extended release formula, Niaspan) has been shown to reduce disease progression in four other clinical trials as well.[1] Good medical doctors will prescribe niacin for reducing cardiovascular disease risk and provide a description of how to use it. Niacin is frequently the gold standard control used for basic research experiments using animal models of atherosclerosis. In clinical trials, when niacin has been compared to other marketed drugs it has led to most undesirable effects for business, but most therapeutically beneficial effects for the fortunate patients. Cardiovascular disease (CVD) kills more individuals than any other disease. Accordingly, there is tremendous drive in the pharmaceutical industry to make drugs. Merck and Schering Plough convinced doctors to spend 21 billion dollars over seven years selling Zetia (ezetimibe). Ultimately however, clinical trials would thereafter reveal that Zetia actually increases cardiovascular events, making mean arterial walls thicker![2] Thus, it is no longer a good business idea for the pharmaceutical industry to compare drugs to niacin head to head. Immediate release (IR) niacin works just as well as prescription extended release (ER) niacin, but it costs approximately fifteen dollars a day to obtain 3 grams, while IR niacin costs just fifty cents. ER niacin causes less of a flush response initially, but with regular usage, IR niacin results in little to no flush at all, while all of the benefits are still reaped.

While the benefits of niacin for treating CVD are undeniable given the rigorously precise biochemical measures, there has been more controversy over the benefits of niacin for treating schizophrenia and behavioral disorders. Sixty years ago, Dr. Abram Hoffer entered this scene at the all-time height of psychiatry equivocation when he first proposed with Dr. Humphry Osmond to try much higher doses of vitamin B_3 for treating what resembled the dementias seen just a decade prior in the pellagra epidemics of the 1940s. Sigmund Freudian-based psychotherapy was all the rage at this time in the early 1950s. "Refrigerator moms" (emotionally unresponsive mothers) were given as the causal explanation for schizophrenia. Abram and Osmond results were stunningly effective in the cure rate for schizophrenia (even more so than today's best medicine used for treating schizophrenia). Nonetheless, poorly understood drugs are repeatedly marketed to suffering schizophrenics, while an increasing variety of other newly defined mental and behavioral disorders are defined. This book, *Niacin: The Real Story*, relates niacin to descriptions of the three main psychotic disorders: bipolar disorder (characterized by dramatic mood swings), schizophrenias (characterized by perceptual hallucinations and delusions), and schizoaffective disorders (characterized by periods of both of these).

As illustrated above with the Zetia example, it has gotten so rare that anyone addresses the most important question anymore: "What works best?" It is such a simple question. Instead, too much research today proceeds primarily from a for-profit motive. It is also so rare to have someone who was around to witness the historical transformation of medical motives from a "health-and-improvement motive" to a "much-increased-profit motive," as Abram Hoffer and Harold Foster did. The profit machine ultimately consumed the spirit or focus of many a well-intentioned doctor, but Abram persisted in weathering the storm, risking his stature among his peers to maintain the premise of his work, always addressing the question: "What works best?" With an open mind and an incredible work ethic, Abram continued following the most recent research right up until the end.

There is so much more to the story of niacin than its success in treating CVD. Firstly, there are other distinct molecular versions of nicotinamide adenine dinucleotide (NAD) precursor besides niacin that are also covered in this book you hold in your hands. Secondly, there are so many observations that would remain hidden from modern medical education if it were not for the work of the author of this book, Dr. Andrew Saul. Abram Hoffer's experiences treating patients with high doses of niacin or niacinamide were almost too numerous to tell.

Even today, niacin, functioning as a precursor to NAD, perennially excites and simulates modern discovery in molecular biology and pharmacology research. One of the most amazing mice used by scientists for twenty-plus years has been the Slow Wallerian Degeneration (Wld[S]) mouse.[3] Wallerian degeneration is the process of neuronal degeneration that occurs after physical insult to the neuron via razor excision or crushing of axons, all in a petri dish. Normal neurons completely degenerate within twenty-four hours of damage; however, the Wld[S] mouse resists degeneration. Amazingly, Wld[S] neurons survive for over two weeks, all without a nucleus, while still being able to be excited for at least a week![4] Eventually the gene was mapped and determined to involve triplication of the NAD-synthesizing enzyme encoded by NMNAT1 (Nicotinamide mononucleotide adenylyltransferase 1), where NAD itself could in part substitute for the neuroprotective activity conferred by this fortunate genetic mutation.[5] Further research realized a role for the NAD-dependent pathways frequently involving histone deacetylase enzyme Sirt1 in Wallerian degeneration, multiple sclerosis, diabetes, Alzheimer's disease, and others in our best animal models available for studying human disease.[6,7] This same Sirt1 enzyme was previously identified as being critical to conferring caloric restriction (CR) dependent increases in lifespan,[8] where CR is the only proven approach shown to consistently extend lifespan in all animal models.

However, with the genome(s) sequenced at the end of the shining day of the molecular biology revolution, the most important question remains: "What works best?" To this day, it would appear that niacin ranks among the highest in this regard. Based on sheer historical observation, pellagra was the most devastating nutritional deficiency epidemic ever reported in the United States of America. This epidemic deficiency was in large part the result of modern developments in food refining, when technological advancements enabled mass milling and the production and introduction of white rice and white flour to large populations of people. The pellagra epidemics followed, and then the golden age of vitamin discovery began. We realize from this history that modern human beings are simply most susceptible to niacin (and vitamin B_1/beriberi) deficiencies. Thus, it simply makes sense that we would most likely benefit from higher dose application of niacin during stress or disease situations, which are well known to actively deplete NAD. Once niacin is transformed to NAD inside the cell, it is used in more biochemical reactions than any other vitamin-derived cofactor (over 450).[9] This surely factors into the molecular basis for its varied physiological activities. Does it not therefore come as little surprise that niacin works to provide relief for so many conditions? Unfortunately, as Abram Hoffer once said, "Niacin works so good that nobody believes it." Reality is what we always want to believe, but sometimes it is hard to believe—the fact is, there truly are so many situations where increased NAD is what we need to allow our body's endogenous chemistry to catch up to the insults inflicted on it—whether it is too much consumption of sugar or alcohol, too much stress, too much fat, and *ad infinitum.*

In basic scientific research, there are many experiments that obviously can never be performed on human beings. We have to learn the tragic way. This involves simple observational analysis, with the most medically significant lessons arising in urgent response to wars rather than through the standard biomedical scientific method. Abram and Harold lived through such wars and worked with the victims, and reported with Andrew Saul on many of these most important examples of treatment with high dose niacin. Their lessons are veritable timeless treasures. Aside from their research, reports of high-dose niacin treatment do not exist in the standard medical education literature. In this book, you will finally observe firsthand examples of the results of clinical niacin use as it has never been told before. It is an invaluable resource for everyone interested in maintaining optimal health.

—W. Todd Penberthy, Ph.D.
Research Professor, University of Central Florida
Department of Molecular Biology and Microbiology

Preface

Many people have no idea how many illnesses are caused by too little niacin, and practically no one realizes just how many illnesses can be cured with megadoses of niacin. It is the authors' intent to change that. Our objective is to provide a reader-friendly, problem-solving book. This book is not nearly so much about the niacin molecule as it is about what can be done with a lot of niacin molecules. Therefore, this book concentrates on niacin's clinical benefits in a number of health conditions. These conditions, successfully treated by pioneering niacin researcher Abram Hoffer, M.D., Ph.D., are based on his more than fifty years of medical practice. Dr. Hoffer, whose capacity for work continually astounded me, began this book at the age of ninety-one. Unfortunately, he died before it was completed. Medical geographer and professor Harry Foster, our coauthor and long-time collaborator, also suffered untimely death during the early stages of writing this work. So, if you wonder why this book is not thicker and more comprehensive, there you have your main reasons. This is most certainly not a textbook. However, standing on the shoulders of these two giants of nutritional science, I have endeavored to add to and complete the existing manuscript without altering Abram's and Harry's voices: Harry, the medical theorist and scholar, and Abram, the experienced and courageous physician and researcher. (You often will find Dr. Hoffer's voice in this book, in first person, with the initials AH following in parentheses.) The other voice is mine (AWS), that of the teacher, raconteur, and parent.

I am honored beyond measure to have worked for years with Dr. Hoffer and Dr. Foster. I think Abram Hoffer and Harry Foster were, and will ever be, regarded as two of the great medical innovators of the modern era. Dr. Hoffer was the world authority on niacin. This constitutes his final work, of which he said, simply: "This book is designed primarily for clinicians and the public who want to learn more and more about niacin and its wonderful properties."

I hope this handbook may prove to be a significant part of his legacy, and of real help to all readers.

—Andrew W. Saul
November 2011

INTRODUCTION
Why Should You Read This Book?

In theory, there is no difference between theory and practice.
In practice there is.
—YOGI BERRA

In *The Structure of Scientific Revolutions*, Thomas Kuhn[1] says that advances in science do not occur in an evolutionary or straight-line manner. Instead, such steps take place in a series of violent revolutions separated by long periods of relative peace. During dramatic uprisings, "one conceptual world view replaces another." These intellectual revolts are not random events. They are promoted by the discovery of significant anomalies: emergent facts that the ruling dominant theory and its supporters fail to adequately explain. These "exceptions to the rule" are the termites of scientific theory. As they multiply, they become more and more difficult to ignore. The newly infected ruling theory weakens until it eventually collapses. A paradigm shift occurs as another takes its place.

While the drug-based pharmaceutical industry continues to control conventional medicine, its support structure is increasingly termite riddled. Weaknesses are being illustrated by new highly critical books, with titles such as *Deadly Medicine*[2], *Overdo$ed America*[3], and *Death by Modern Medicine*[4]. Of course, the drug-based approach to health will not be abandoned any time soon unless society has a viable alternative, waiting, like an understudy, in the wings. There it must be quietly attracting its own, more open-minded supporters.

The authors of this book are members of one such group: advocates of orthomolecular (nutrition-based) medicine. They support an approach to human wellness that involves the use, not of drugs, but of substances that naturally occur in the human body.[5] Niacin is one of these, and as such seems destined to eventually play a significant role in the upcoming, inevitable medical paradigm shift. It is impossible here to show all the advantages society will gain by switching to nutrition-based medicine. However, this initial chapter provides a variety of examples drawn from several specific categories of wellness. The remainder of the book seeks to examine, in much more detail, the case that can be made for the far more widespread use of one such nutrient, niacin, for the prevention and treatment of health issues.

By eating diets that are deficient in essential nutrients, many individuals trigger their own chronic degenerative diseases later in life. It has been known for millennia that the basis for health is good nutrition. Orthomolecular medicine, a description coined in 1968 by Linus Pauling,[6] goes further. Pauling describes a medical modality that uses nutrients and normal (that is, "ortho") constituents of the body in specific optimum quantities as the dominant treatment. Such health-nutritional relationships have been comprehensively explored most recently by Hoffer and Saul in *Orthomolecular Medicine for Everyone: Megavitamin Therapeutics for Families and Physicians*[7].

It has been further recognized that individuals are unique in their daily requirements for vitamins, minerals, or protein.[8] For *each* nutrient, at least 2.5 percent will need higher levels than the rest of the population. There are about three dozen nutrients. Doing the math, it becomes apparent that most people are deficient in something—even if they consume USRDA (United States Recommended Dietary Allowance) nutrient levels every day.

We are all different, and you are a bit different every day. Illness, medications, age, variations in diet, fatigue, and stress are among the many factors that today can make you different from the you of yesterday. It has been said that you are what you eat. This very orthomolecular concept is

---

"Orthomolecular" means the right or the correct molecule. The name was coined by Linus Pauling in 1968. Conventional pharmaceuticals tend to be "toximolecular." Vitamins and insulin are examples of orthomolecular therapeutic substances. Chemotherapy would be an example of a toximolecular therapy.

true. But, in a deeper way, you are what you absorb. To illustrate, as Hoffer and Saul point out:

> In regard to nutrients, there may be a problem with absorption in the intestine. Thus with pernicious anemia, specific areas in the gut that normally absorb vitamin B_{12} are lacking, or after the vitamin is absorbed it may not be combined effectively into its coenzyme, or it may be wasted or held too tenaciously by some organ system, thus depriving other parts of the body.[9]

We need all the nutrients all the time, in the same way that an aircraft needs all its wheels and wings. Roger Williams[10] has described a basic concept called the "orchestra principal." Just as it is impossible to claim that one instrument in an orchestra is more important than another, so to maintain health, all the nutrients required by the body must be available to ensure well-being. Though impossible to outline the enormous number of illnesses that can develop as a result of nutritional imbalance, we can illustrate the principle. It seems likely that calcium and selenium deficiencies promote many cancers,[11] excess aluminum and inadequate magnesium and calcium are linked to Alzheimer's disease,[12] and a lack of sulfur is associated with osteoarthritis.[13] Certainly there are many other well-known nutrition-illness connections as well.

As will be seen from the remainder of this book, niacin plays an especially significant role in orthomolecular medicine. Inevitably, its use will increase as the medical paradigm shift occurs. Orthomolecular treatments are typically far less expensive than drug-based conventional protocols. Embracing orthomolecular treatments will make prevention and treatment available to the poor. If this statement might seem overly ambitious, we might consider this: a single orange may cost one dollar. It would provide about 50 milligrams (mg) of vitamin C. A bottle of 100 tablets of vitamin C, 500 mg each, costs about five dollars. In terms of vitamin content, the orange gives you 50 mg per dollar. The supplement gives you 10,000 mg per dollar. There are of course other nutritional factors and advantages to eating oranges, such as sugars, taste, bioflavinoids, and fiber. However, one cannot easily deny, at least in terms of vitamin C, that the supplement is 200 times cheaper, costing about half a cent for the amount of vitamin C in a one-dollar orange. Even if your oranges could cost only one-tenth as much, an impossible ten cents each, the supplement is still twenty times cheaper.

The same is true for niacin. Niacin supplements cost approximately five dollars for 100 tablets of 250 mg each. That works out to be about 5,000 mg niacin per dollar. Healthy foods naturally containing significant amounts of niacin cost far more. Once again, the many nutritional advantages of eating kidneys, liver, whole-grain bread, nuts, and green leafy vegetables are considerable and undeniable. In terms of niacin content, however, there is no competition. Several dollars' worth of these foods provides only tens of milligrams of niacin. Niacin-fortified foods such as breakfast cereals, white bread, and pasta are slightly cheaper niacin sources, but not much. Interestingly, the fact that milled grains have any niacin at all is due to niacin being added to them in the manufacturing process. Adding niacin to foods is a form of low-dose supplementation.

The USRDA, which is far too low, is less than 18 mg. Yet bodily need for niacin varies with activity, body size, and illness.[14] About half of all Americans will not get even the RDA amount of niacin from their diets. Niacin's special importance is indicated in that the US RDA for niacin, which again we say is a very low figure, is actually twenty or more times higher than the RDA for other B vitamins. Twenty teaspoons will not clean up after a hurricane much faster than one will. We think that a lack of sufficient niacin is a real and continuing public health problem.

CHAPTER 1

What Is Niacin?

*For every drug that benefits a patient, there is a natural
substance that can achieve the same effect.*
—CARL C. PFEIFFER, M.D., PH.D.

Niacin is a small molecule, smaller than the simplest sugar, glucose. Niacin is made of only fourteen atoms. ($C_6H_5NO_2$). How can just one molecule have such profound effects on health?

Niacin is one of the members of a family of substances involved in the pyridine nucleotide cycle. It plays a role in over 500 reactions in the body. Interfering with any of these vital reactions will cause disease and, conversely, improving and restoring these reactions will be therapeutic.

Why, then, is the medical profession so ignorant of this vitamin and its vast importance? In 2011, a Google search will hit (find a match on) "niacin" about 4 million times. For comparison, Haldol, one of the first antipsychotics, had 700,000 hits; Zyprexa, nearly 8 million hits; Prozac, over 13 million hits; and Effexor, close to 10 million hits. The four antipsychotics have been advertised and promoted with multimillion dollar budgets, while niacin has not been promoted at all, except by a very few physicians who found its properties so valuable. There are few advertisements in medical journals from niacin manufacturers. Niacin is still advocated by word of mouth.

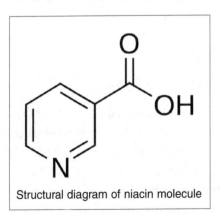

Structural diagram of niacin molecule

Drugs are heavily advertised in both the medical journals and in the popular press. They have to be: it takes a lot of public persuasion to promote products that are rarely effective and carry with them danger-ous side effects, including death. The major side effect of niacin is longer life.

It is obviously impossible to describe everything that is known about niacin. This would require an encyclopedia. In this book, we will concen-trate on its clinical aspects and on conditions that one of us, Abram Hof-fer (AH), found were helped in over fifty years of psychiatric practice.

OR MORE CORRECTLY, WHAT ARE *THEY*?

Niacin's original chemical name was nicotinic acid. The name was changed to niacin to remove confusion with nicotine. Niacin was also known early on as vitamin B_3, since it was the third water-soluble vitamin to be iden-tified. Normally, this term would have been eliminated once its chemical structure had been determined, but it was brought back by Bill W., cofounder of Alcoholics Anonymous (AA), who wanted a catchy name he could use to inform members of AA about its immense value for the treat-ment of alcohol addicts. There is a question whether it should have been classed with the vitamins because it can be made in the body from tryp-tophan and is used by the body in quantities more appropriate to amino acids. It has been suggested that it should be classed as an amino acid, but it is now too late to do anything about this.

Gutierrez[1] outlined a study at the University of California at Irvine which showed that liver cells in vitro treated with niacin did not take up as much HDL, which could explain why it increased HDL in blood. This may be the first explanation of why niacin is so effective. But it also shows that niacin is not toxic to live cells. This should help quell the delusion held by so many doctors that niacin is liver toxic.

Forms of Niacin and How They Differ in Action

Derivatives of niacin (nicotinic acid) have been examined for their ability to alter lipid levels as well as niacin does. It would be advantageous to many if the niacin vasodilatation (flush) were eliminated or removed.

Niacin lowers cholesterol, elevates high-density lipoprotein (HDL) cho-lesterol, and reduces the ravages of heart disease, but causes flushing when it is first taken. The flushing reaction dissipates in time and in most cases is gone or very minor within a matter of weeks. Niacinamide, which is not a vasodilator, does not produce a flush, but it has no effect on blood fats (lipids). Inositol hexaniacinate will lower cholesterol without the flushing side effect, but does not do so as well as plain niacin.

	NIACIN	NIACINAMIDE	INOSITOL HEXANIACINATE	SUSTAINED RELEASE (HARD TABLET)	EXTENDED/TIME RELEASE
Blood Lipid Benefits	Yes	No	Yes	Yes	Yes
Psychiatric Benefits	Yes	Yes	Yes	Yes	Yes
Flush	Yes	No	No	Sometimes	No
Nausea at Several Thousand mg/day	No	Yes	No	No	No
Highest Degree of Liver Safety	Yes	Yes	Yes	No	No
Complete Tablet Dissolution	Yes	Yes	Yes	No	Yes

Niacin

Both niacin and niacinamide are effective against mental illness. Both will prevent and treat simple nutritional deficiency. Niacin (but not niacinamide) taken in high doses will produce a skin flush in most people. This is why niacinamide is the much more common form used in multiple vitamins and other dietary supplements. Unlike many other vitamins, all forms of niacin are exceptionally stable and each has a very long shelf life. The vitamin is not harmed by heat.

Several formulations are available to decrease the intensity of the niacin vasodilatation or flush. The best known is called "no-flush" niacin and is available over-the-counter. It is an inositol derivative with six niacin molecules attached to each benzene ring. There are other flushless forms available by prescription only, but they are much more expensive. Billions have been spent trying to find something as good as niacin that can be patented. This is a major waste of money and time, since the best anti-flush preparation is niacin itself. Most people stop flushing with continued use. The best antidote to the flush is an informed patient and doctor. As Dr. William Parsons Jr. wrote, "A doctor must know niacin in order to use it."

Another major difference between niacin and niacinamide is that niacin normalizes blood lipid values. It lowers low-density lipoprotein cholesterol ("bad" cholesterol), elevates high-density cholesterol ("good" cholesterol), lowers triglycerides, lowers lipoprotein(a) [Lp(a) is considered a risk factor for heart disease], and lowers the anti-inflammatory factor C-reactive protein. It therefore is the best substance known for these important therapeutic effects. Niacinamide has none of these properties.

Niacinamide

The other common form of niacin is nicotinamide, known more commonly as niacinamide. Both niacin and niacinamide forms are precursors to the active anti-pellagra factor NAD (nicotinamide adenine dinucleotide). A third form of vitamin B_3, nicotinamide riboside, was discovered in 2004, and little is known about it. Your body uses NAD (with a hydrogen, it is NADH) in over 450 biochemical reactions, most of which are involved in anabolic and catabolic reactions. Most people tend to associate NAD with glycolysis (sugar breakdown) and ATP (energy production). However, NAD is involved with many other reactions as a cofactor, including either the synthesis (anabolism) or the breakdown (catabolism) of just about every molecule our cells make: steroids, prostaglandins, and enzymes. NAD is involved in cell signaling and assists in ongoing repair of your DNA. There are several important reactions where it functions as a substrate for the enzymes PARP, Sirtuin, and IDO.[2,3,4]

Niacin and niacinamide have different properties. The most commonly observed difference is that when niacin is first taken, it causes a flush that starts in the forehead and travels down the body with varying intensities. Niacinamide does this very rarely. If there is a flush from niacinamide, it is very unpleasant.

Niacinamide is more likely to cause nausea at long-term, medium-high dosages than are the other forms of B_3. By medium high, we mean several thousand mg per day. Niacin and inositol hexaniacinate generally do not cause nausea unless the dose is extremely high, on the order of tens of thousands of mg per day. No one would need to take that excessive amount of B_3, and no one should. And just to be sure, nausea indicates overdose. On the other hand, niacinamide has been successfully used at maintained doses of several thousand mg per day by Dr. William Kaufman to treat arthritis (see Chapter 7). He reported virtually zero side effects.

Inositol Hexaniacinate

For those few who can not tolerate niacin, there is the option of using inositol hexaniacinate. This preparation has most of the therapeutic advantages of niacin and none of the side effects. It is available in health food stores as "no-flush niacin." It costs perhaps three times as much as "regular" niacin, but this is still much better than the cheapest statins (the most expensive costs a fortune). Drug coverage plans should cover inositol hexaniacinate as they now cover niacin to achieve some of this savings and, even more important, improve the health of their patients.[5,6]

Inositol hexaniacinate is an ester of inositol and nicotinic acid. It is sometimes called inositol hexanicotinate. Each inositol molecule contains six nicotinic acid molecules. This ester is broken down slowly in the body. It is about as effective as nicotinic acid and is almost free of side effects. There is very little flushing, gastrointestinal distress, or other side effects. Inositol, considered one of the lesser-important B vitamins, does have a function in the body as a messenger molecule and may add something to the therapeutic properties of the nicotinic acid. The name "nicotinic" is often confusing. Remember that niacin (nicotinic acid) and nicotine have no physiological properties in common.

I (AH) used this compound for thirty years for patients who can not or will not tolerate the flush. It is very gentle, effective, and can be tolerated by almost every person who uses it.

Extended-Release, Sustained-Release, or Time-Release Niacin?

Get ready to be confused a bit: these terms are often used interchangeably. Sometimes "sustained release," "time release," or "extended release" niacin is simply inositol hexaniacinate, discussed above. Sustained-release, time-release, and extended-release niacin may also refer to physical or chemical tableting variations of regular niacin, generally either a hard-matrix tablet or coated little pellets in a tablet or capsule. It is a perfectly good idea: If a vitamin tablet physically dissolves slowly, there is a sustained-release effect. Extended-release and time-release are very similar: release is chemically delayed. The goal of all these preparations is a reduced niacin "flush." (We further discuss the niacin flush in Chapter 4.)

Sensitive persons sometimes report that the harder matrix of some sustained-release tablets can be felt in the stomach. Taking sustained-release tablets with a meal or snack may help reduce this sensation. Hard-matrix sustained release tablets are the most likely to fail to break down in the digestive tract of elderly people. In other words, one may not be getting what the label claims, not because it isn't in the tablet, but because the tablet never digests completely enough to release it.

Sustained-, extended-, and time-release niacin are often advertised as not causing a flush at all. This claim may not be completely true; some-times the flush is just postponed. It may be difficult to determine your optimum level with an extended-, sustained-, or time-release product. All three are also more costly. But the biggest reason to avoid sustained-release niacin is that relatively more reports of side effects stem from use of that form.[7] A 2007 review by Guyton and Bays of many niacin therapy stud-ies reveals that regular ("immediate release," or IR) niacin is quite safe; extended- or time-release are safe, but unnecessarily pricey, and sustained-release (SR) has the most side effects. They write:

> Shortly after Altschul and colleagues described cholesterol lowering by niacin in 1955, sustained-release (SR) formulations were developed in an attempt to reduce flushing. However, these were quickly found to be hepatotoxic in some patients. . . . Henkin et al.[19] found 8 cases of hepatitis in 15 patients using SR niacin, compared with none in 67 patients using regular niacin. Three patients who had experienced hepatitis with SR niacin were subsequently able to tolerate equal or higher doses of regular niacin.[20] McKenney et al.[3] directly compared IR and SR niacin in a randomized clinical trial with dosage escalation from 500 to 3,000 mg/day over a period of 30 weeks. None of the 23 patients taking IR niacin developed hepatotoxic effects, whereas 12 of 23 patients (52%) taking SR niacin did. The increase in liver tox-icity with SR niacin mainly occurred with doses 1,500 mg/day.[8] [Cita-tions numbered as in original source.[9]]

We therefore prefer and recommend manual, divided doses of regular, immediate-release niacin, not sustained-release niacin. For those who sim-ply must avoid the flush, the alternative forms of niacin are acceptable.

NADH Supplements

NADH (nicotinamide adenine dinucleotide, plus hydrogen) is an antioxi-dant coenzyme, an activated form of niacin. It is involved in cellular energy production. It has been available in a stabilized form as a dietary supplement since the mid-1990s. NADH is extremely costly per milligram (mg), but only a few mg are normally taken. It is claimed to help with chronic fatigue and other energy-related disorders, and perhaps Alzheimer's disease, Parkinson's disease, and depression. Since NADH is naturally and continually made in your body from niacin, we think taking a lot of niacin is a far cheaper therapy. Niacinamide also increases the body's own production of NADH. NADH research is promising but not definitive. Niacin has a longer, and stronger, track record of effectiveness. We also think that, generally speaking, vitamin C is a much cheaper way to get antioxidant benefits.

Tryptophan

All forms of vitamin B$_3$ are anti-pellagra, all are precursors of NAD, are available commercially, and all have major therapeutic properties beyond what most people expect from their nutritional, anti-pellagra properties. Tryptophan is also a precursor to NAD. However, at high doses, tryptophan may have health concerns. Tryptophan has been connected with eosinophilia-myalgia syndrome, characterized by elevated white blood cell levels and muscle pain. The connection may be due primarily to manufacturing error with genetically-engineered materials. However, limited plasma tryptophan plays key roles in limiting a potentially hyperactive immune system. Thus, tryptophan is not generally taken as a precursor to NAD.

Other "Niacins"

One may occasionally come across what may be described as other forms of niacin. These include xanthinol niacinate (or xanthinol nicotinate), nicotinyl alcohol, ciclonicate, and etofylline nicotinate. All are vasodilators, which means they cause blood vessels to expand slightly. Nicotinyl alcohol also lowers cholesterol. Are these "designer niacins" worth seeking out and paying for? Maybe, maybe not. When niacin and xanthinol nicotinate were compared in a double-blind experiment, it was found that niacin "treatment resulted in improvement of sensory register and short-term memory, while xanthinol nicotinate improved sensory register, short-term memory and long-term memory. In comparison with placebo, both active compounds yielded improvements of 10–40%."[10] Xanthinol niacinate seemed to work better in elderly subjects.

However, xanthinol is a derivative of theophylline, a molecule that resembles caffeine and is present in tea and cocoa leaves. Theophylline is a central nervous system stimulant with properties similar to caffeine. It is therefore questionable whether the active part is the niacin or the xanthinol. Ciclonicate is a drug that was abandoned in the mid-1980s. It is still available outside the United States. Nothing has been published about it in twenty-six years. We would not consider these as forms of niacin, regardless what may be claimed by promoters.

Chromium polynicotinate (or chromium polyniacinate) is a chromium supplement that contains niacin. It is also known as "niacin-bound chromium." There have been several studies that have shown niacin-bound chromium may be more effective in increasing insulin sensitivity, improving glucose tolerance, and reducing excess body fat than other forms of chromium. Niacin-bound chromium has also been reported to help lower cholesterol and systolic blood pressure.[11–14] It may be that some of chromium's claims to fame are not so much due to niacin enhancing the biochemical delivery of chromium but are actually due to chromium enhancing the delivery of niacin. (We will discuss niacin in cardiovascular disease in Chapter 10.)

What About Niacin in Foods?

Many foods contain a little niacin. None contain therapeutic quantities. Foods relatively high in niacin include lean meat, fish, organ meats (kidney, liver), clams, shrimp, pork, dairy products, nuts and seeds, wheat germ, whole wheat products, beans, and green leafy vegetables. So is it enough to just eat more of them? Unfortunately, no. Even an ideal diet, very heavy in all of these nutritious foods, will not come close to even a 100 mg niacin supplement. We need extra niacin.

CHAPTER 2

How Niacin Therapy Began

*People's minds are changed through observation
and not through argument.*

—WILL ROGERS

A deficiency is present when the very small amounts of nutrients that are needed to keep one going in the usual common state of poor health are not present in the diet. Most of the people living in North America can not get enough vitamins and trace minerals from their food and therefore are suffering from various degrees of micronutrient deficiency. The daily recommended doses established by government are grounded in deficiency. They are derived from the old vitamins-as-prevention paradigm, now 100 years old, and ignore the modern vitamins-as-treatment paradigm. The classical deficiency diseases are beriberi, pellagra, scurvy, rickets, and pernicious anemia.

PELLAGRA (VITAMIN B₃ DEFICIENCY) AND SCHIZOPHRENIA (VITAMIN B₃ DEPENDENCY)

After Dr. Joseph Goldberger discovered the cause of pellagra, a deficiency disease, and Dr. Conrad Elvehjem in Wisconsin discovered that niacin and niacinamide were the anti-pellagra vitamins, pellagra was vanquished. The timely mandatory fortification of white flour in 1942 by the United States government during the Second World War saved humanity incalculable numbers of lives and disability and trillions of dollars in costs. This brilliant decision may have even influenced the outcome of the war.

In 1930, 30,000 Americans died from pellagra in the southeast United States. Pellagra is characterized by the four D's: dermatitis, diarrhea, dementia, and death. The dementia or psychosis associated with pellagra can not be differentiated on clinical grounds alone. It can be readily distinguished by the nutritional history and the use of vitamin B_3 as a diagnostic test. If patients given niacin recovered in a few days or weeks, they were diagnosed as having pellagra. If it took a lot longer or did not occur because too little was given, they were diagnosed as schizophrenic. This was the style of diagnosis by pellagrologists in the United States in the mid-1930s once niacin/niacinamide was identified as the anti-pellagra vitamin.

The major difference is that pellagra is caused by total malnutrition generated by a diet high in corn and non-nutritious food, while in schizophrenia, the major deficiency is vitamin B_3 in most cases where starvation is not endemic. The skin lesions in pellagra are responsive to tryptophan. Like pellagrins, schizophrenic patients exposed to the sun suffered skin pigment changes. The pellagrologists in the 1930s and 1940s were very good observers. How could they miss this obvious similarity between schizophrenia and pellagra? They did not miss it. But they were so indoctrinated by the vitamins-as-prevention paradigm that they were blinded by theory rather than guided by what they observed. They knew pellagra was a deficiency disease and that only small amounts were needed to cure and to prevent further relapses in most cases. They knew schizophrenia was a major intractable chronic mental disease. Because they were blinded by the old vitamin paradigm, they insisted the two were different conditions. When niacin became available, they gave it to both pellagrins and schizophrenic patients. According to their definition, they were pellagrins if they responded in a short period of time, even if it took 1,000 mg daily. They remained schizophrenic if they did not respond at these doses. The pellagrinologists were unable to make the differential diagnosis on clinical grounds alone. And because these experts were so certain the diseases were not the same, investigators thereafter would no longer examine the issue.

How Dr. Hoffer Became Involved with Niacin

I (AH) looked on niacin as a drug, as did the FDA, and not as a vitamin. Only much later did I realize what we were dealing with. The vitamin-as-prevention paradigm was enshrined around the following beliefs: (1) vitamins are needed only to prevent the classical well-known deficiency

Joseph Goldberger, M.D. (1874–1929)

Orthomolecular Medicine Hall of Fame, 2008

Goldberger is my model of
a brilliant scientist.
—ABRAM HOFFER, M.D., PH.D.

Joseph Goldberger was born in 1874 and studied medicine at Bellevue Hospital Medical School in New York, graduating with honors in 1895. After an internship at Bellevue Hospital College, he engaged in private practice for two years and then joined the Public Health Service Corps in 1899. During routine work as a quarantine officer on Ellis Island, Goldberger rapidly acquired a reputation for outstanding investigative studies of various infectious diseases, including yellow fever, dengue fever, and typhus. Goldberger devoted the latter part of his career to studying pellagra. After quickly contradicting the contemporary general belief that pellagra was an infectious disease, he spent the last fifteen years of his life trying to prove that its cause was a dietary deficiency. During the first half of the twentieth century, an epidemic of pellagra produced roughly 3 million cases in the United States, about 100,000 of which were fatal.[1]

Abram Hoffer adds: "In the early 1940s, the United States government mandated the addition of niacinamide to flour. This eradicated the terrible pandemic of pellagra in just two years, and ought to be recognized as the most successful public health measure for the elimination of a major disease in psychiatry, the pellagra psychoses. The reaction of contemporary physicians was predictable. Indeed, at the time, Canada rejected the idea and declared the addition of vitamins to flour to be an adulteration. The United States has long been the leading nation in nutrition research."

Knowledge comes at a cost: Goldberger had yellow fever, dengue, and very nearly died of typhus. According to the U.S. National Institutes of Health, he "stepped on Southern pride when he linked the poverty of Southern sharecroppers, tenant farmers, and mill workers to the deficient diet that caused pellagra."[2]

In the end, Goldberger was nominated for the Nobel Prize. Had he not died earlier in the year, he might well have shared it with vitamin researchers Christiaan Eijkman and Frederick G. Hopkins in 1929.

Alan Kraut's prize-winning book, *Goldberger's War: The Life and Work of a Public Health Crusader* is an excellent source on this outstanding pioneer.

diseases; and (2) Only very small doses, the usual vitamin doses, are needed. It followed that one should not give vitamins unless these deficiency diseases were present and large doses were not needed and were forbidden. Giving large doses of niacin to schizophrenic patients broke every rule of the vitamin-as-prevention paradigm. Had the pellagrologists properly determined the optimum dosage for the B vitamins on a large scale and not been blinded by the vitamin-as-prevention paradigm, we might have had a treatment for schizophrenia much earlier.

COMPARISON OF SCHIZOPHRENIC AND PELLAGRA PSYCHOSIS		
	SCHIZOPHRENIA	PELLAGRA
Perceptual		
Visual	Yes	Yes
Auditory	Yes	Yes
Others	Yes	Yes
Thought disorder	Yes	Yes
Mood disorder	Yes	Yes
Behavior changes	Yes	Yes
Skin pigmentation	Yes-minor	Yes-major
Gastrointestinal	Yes-minor	Yes-major
Deaths increased	Yes	Yes
Reasons	Heart; Malnutrition	Suicide
Treatment	Diet	Diet
	Niacin 3,000 mg and up	Niacin 100 to 1,000 mg
Time required	Months to years	Months

The adrenochrome (oxidized adrenaline) hypothesis of Hoffer, Osmond, and Smythies in 1954 suggested that any decrease in the production of adrenalin would be therapeutic for schizophrenic patients, as this would decrease the amount of this catechol that could be converted into adrenochrome. Niacin is one of the major methyl acceptors in the body, and it was possible that by depleting methyl groups, less noradrenalin would be converted into adrenalin. Niacin was safe, could be taken forever, and protected against pellagra, a recent scourge of mankind. It had remarkable antipsychotic effects with the pellagra psychosis, so it became reasonable to test its effect on schizophrenic patients. In 1952 I did not realize that the pellagra psychosis was identical with the schizophrenic psychosis. Our first pilot trials were very successful. We followed these with a small series of double-blind, randomized, placebo-controlled, prospective studies on nonchronic patients, the first in psychiatric history. We doubled the two-year recovery rate to 75 percent compared to 35 percent for the placebo. Once you have see schizophrenic patients become normal, it remains unforgettable. These controlled studies have been confirmed by a large number of clinical open studies, through my own experience in treating well over 5,000 patients since 1952, and in one NIMH-sponsored double-blind controlled trial by Wittenborn in 1974.[3]

CHAPTER 3

How Niacin Works, and Why We Need More of It

Half of what we will teach you is wrong.
The problem is, we don't know which half.
—DR ABRAM HOFFER, QUOTING ONE OF HIS MEDICAL SCHOOL
PROFESSORS ON THE FIRST DAY OF CLASS

For many biological variables, if one charts the number of individuals having a characteristic against its frequency in the population, the curve on the chart follows a so-called normal distribution form. For example, if one measures the height of men, there will be a range between a low figure to a high figure, but the majority of men will be somewhere in the middle. More men will be five foot ten than five feet tall, and fewer will be six foot ten than five foot ten. Almost all biological variables have this variation. The curve is a bell-shaped curve, and most of the values will lie within two standard deviations from the mean. The same distribution applies to our need for nutrients.

Roger J. Williams made it very clear in his writing about biochemical individuality that we are not alike and we do differ in this way. We have different needs for calories, for example, and of course for nutrients, which are so essential. But the optimum needs for vitamins have not been determined. I do not know of any study where the optimum needs for vitamin C have been determined. The vitamin-as-prevention paradigm has been the major obstruction to this research. It forced everyone to accept that vitamins were needed only in very small amounts. It limited examination of needs to individuals who required lower amounts than the average by excluding the needs of those of us who required much more. The vitamin-as-treatment paradigm broke this rule and forced serious examination of the population who required much more no matter what the reasons were. It is known that disease, stress, and many other factors determine how much of a nutrient is needed, and this is not a static figure.

Let us assume that the most reasonable hypothesis is, if one measured the optimum nutrient requirements of a large population, it would follow the same bell-shaped curve as most other biological variables. The individuals in this population would not be well unless they received whatever was their own optimum requirement. The current Recommended Dietary Allowances (RDAs) are based on very little good research done so many years ago and enforced by legal action that did not take this important hypothesis into account.

Once the mean optimum value had been determined, one would expect that people consuming values on the low side of the value would not be as healthy as people taking the mean value. The further from the mean these individuals were, the sicker they would be. If they were two standard deviations away from the mean, they would develop pellagra, the niacin deficiency disease. The closer they were to the mean optimum intake (MOI), the healthier they would be.

If one could depend only upon the natural amount of the vitamin in food, it would be easier to meet one's nutritional requirements and much less attention would have to be paid to the quality of the diet. The optimum dose is that which meets the physiological needs of a particular person without side effects. When dealing with vitamins, taking more than the optimum requirement is not harmful unless enormous doses are taken. This is in striking contrast with pharmaceutical drugs, where taking too much is much more harmful than taking too little.

Just the opposite is true with vitamins. Taking too little is more harmful than taking too much—again within reason. Any substance—no matter how safe—will have side effects if the amount is much too great. Thus, if vitamin C is taken in large doses, it will cause diarrhea in some people. This is not necessarily toxic, but if the diarrhea is excessive it might be. Therefore, the onset of diarrhea is used as an indicator that the person has reached the upper end point of how much vitamin C he or she should take. This is known as the sublaxative level. Ideally, we should talk about the relative deficiency of a nutrient in a particular person. If a person needs 1,000 mg (milligrams) of vitamin C each day and eats only 100 mg, his intake will be 10 percent of his optimum needs. If he or she needs 100 mg daily and gets only 30 mg, that person is getting only 30 percent of his or her optimum needs. Taking more than the optimum is of little value but as it is not dangerous; it is better to err on the side of a little too much rather than risk deficiency. The only waste will be in the cost of the vitamin and fortunately, as they are not patented, their costs have not jetted into the stratosphere.

WHY DO WE NEED MORE NIACIN?

Subjects who do not get enough vitamin B$_3$ because of their diet will get pellagra. Patients whose vitamin B$_3$ requirements are in the upper range will never get enough through their diet, and they will have to use supplements. They are the vitamin dependent group. The range of vitamin B$_3$ requirements varies from the left end of the bell-shaped curve to the group who need a lot more at the right end of the requirement distribution. We believe that half or more of our population needs vitamin B$_3$ supplementation.

Fetal Development and Future Diseases

A woman's diet during pregnancy has very significant ramifications on her fetus.[1] This, of course, has been known for millennia. Much more recently, however, it has been demonstrated that nutrition is the number-one intra-uterine environmental variable that alters expression of the fetal genome.[2] As a result of its impact on the genes of the fetus, what a mother eats has lifelong consequences for her child. To illustrate, her diet can greatly alter the risk of her offspring for developing specific diseases in adulthood, a phenomenon known as "fetal programming." Optimal maternal nutrition, therefore, can both promote healthy fetal growth and lower the risk of her child experiencing various chronic diseases in adulthood.[3]

In some regions, soils and potable water are so deficient in a specific mineral(s) that certain infant abnormalities are commonplace and said to be endemic. Iodine deficiency, for example, which interferes with the normal production and regulation of thyroid hormones, is associated with a spectrum of deficits ranging from cretinism, hypothyroidism, and dwarfishness to deafness.[4] Endemic abnormalities triggered by maternal iodine deficiency occur in 1,550 Chinese regions.[5] Extreme selenium deficiency is also experienced in parts of China, resulting in endemic diseases such as Keshan disease, an endemic cardiomyopathy, and Kaschin-Beck disease, an endemic osteoarthropathy.[6]

Intrauterine environmental nutritional deficiencies can alter the expression [development] of the fetal genome with specific lifelong consequences.[7] It has been suggested, for example, that fetal iodine deficiency may result in an abnormally high requirement of dopamine, which, in adulthood, increases the risk of illnesses such as Parkinson's disease and multiple sclerosis.[8,9] This phenomenon is termed "fetal programming" and has led to the belief that there are often "fetal origins of adult disease."[10]

Nutrition and Genetic Individuality

Consider that chimpanzees are more than 98 percent genetically identical to humans. What a difference that other 2 percent makes, eh?

Genes are blueprints that permit the production of proteins. These in turn are needed to create, among other things, enzymes. Nevertheless, slight differences in specific genes, called alleles, occur from one person to the next. As a result, many genes carry two, several, or even many variants of the same genetic information. Accordingly, even members of the same family may have distinct genetic information in specific genes. While some of these minor genetic differences cause almost insignificant variations in information and do not significantly affect well-being, others can have profound negative impacts.[11]

A study published by Dr. Robert Ames and coworkers in the *American Journal of Clinical Nutrition* points out that "The proportion of mutations in a disease gene that is responsive to high concentrations of a vitamin or substrate may be one-third or greater."[12] Roughly one-third of such genetic mutations appear to create enzymes that have very decreased binding activities for their coenzymes. This results in an enzyme that is less reactive than normal, making the human carrier of this polymorphism more susceptible to health problems associated with an inadequacy in the enzyme involved.

Genes are not destiny, however. As Ames and colleagues explain:

> About 50 human genetic diseases due to defective enzymes can be remedied or ameliorated by the administration of high doses of the vitamin component of the corresponding coenzyme, which at least partially restores enzymatic activity. Several single-nucleotide polymorphisms, in which the variant amino acid reduces coenzyme binding and thus enzymatic activity, are likely to be remediable by raising cellular concentrations of the cofactor through high-dose vitamin therapy.[13]

Simply put, there are numerous people who carry genetic mutations that mean they must eat diets that are unusually elevated in a particular nutrient. If they eat a normal diet, they cannot produce effective levels of the enzyme activity required for health. As a result, they will inevitably begin to develop the associated deficiency disease. For people carrying certain alleles, very high intakes of vitamin or mineral supplements are not a health threat or a fad—they are the only way they can remain healthy. In some cases, they require as much as one thousand or more times the Recommended Daily Allowance of a particular nutrient.

Ames and colleagues provided details of many of such coenzyme-decreased binding affinity disorders and the nutrients that are likely to ameliorate them.[14] One example is the enzyme cystathionine b-synthase, which catalyzes homocysteine and serine, creating cystalthionine. People who have a defective form of this enzyme cannot do this and, as a consequence, have abnormally high blood and urine homocysteine levels. These are known to be associated with numerous health problems including mental retardation, vascular and skeletal defects, and optic lens dislocation. In approximately 50 percent of cystathinonine b-synthase deficient patients, very high doses of vitamin B_6 can provide significant improvement by lowering the homocysteine and serine concentrations to normal levels.[15]

Nutrients and Infectious Diseases

Humans have evolved very complex immune systems to protect themselves against infection by a wide variety of pathogens. Conversely, pathogens possess a diverse genetic versatility that permits them to mutate and so escape such population immunity.[16] These conflicting host-pathogen objectives have lead to an evolutionary "arms race." In this battle for supremacy, pathogens typically seek to deplete their hosts of specific nutrients that are necessary for the functioning of the human immune system. Once infection occurs, the pathogen continues to rob its host of the same nutrient(s), often causing many of the disease symptoms and sequela [negative aftereffects].[17]

This means that specific diets and supplements can greatly reduce the risk of infection by a particular pathogen. Even after this "invasion" has occurred, the same nutrients may help to hasten disease recovery and reduce its severity. Numerous examples of these relationships are apparent in the literature. To illustrate, in malaria, Plasmodium falciparum competes with its host for vitamin A.[18] In some cases, an extreme deficiency of this vitamin leads to blindness. Plasmodium falciparum also abstracts zinc[19] from its host. Interestingly, 200,000 International Units of vitamin A, given to children four times a year, can greatly lower susceptibility to malaria.[20] It is clearly both a promising preventative and treatment for the disease. In contrast, infection by the Coxsackie B virus seems to result in a selenium deficiency because this pathogen encodes for an analogue of glutathione peroxidase. This trace mineral deficiency-viral infection has been associated with both myocardial infarction[21] and Keshan disease. As suggested here, selenium supplementation can cause dramatic drops in the incidence of Keshan disease.[22] It also lowers heart attack risk, reducing reinfarction rates.[23] HIV-1 also depletes its host of the four nutrients required to make the selenoenzyme glutathione peroxidase. As a result, those infected slowly become deficient in selenium and the three amino acids: cysteine, glutamine, and tryptophan. These deficiencies cause major symptoms that together are called AIDS.[24] Open and closed African trials involving high doses of these four nutrients have shown that the correct nutritional supplements can reverse the symptoms of AIDS and prevent HIV-positive patients from developing this disease.[25] It is apparent, therefore, that the supplementation of diet with specific nutrients, including vitamins, minerals, and amino acids, can reduce infection by numerous pathogens. Beyond this, when infection still takes place, the use of such nutrients to treat the resulting illness may prevent or reverse many of the symptoms and sequela commonly associated with diseases as different as malaria, myocardial infarction, Keshan disease, and HIV/AIDS.

Supplements and Longevity

Recent research has shown that there may be an important link between life expectancy and the use of vitamins. The June 2009 issue of the *American Journal of Clinical Nutrition* includes evidence that multivitamin supplements may prolong lifespan by reducing the speed with which telomeres shorten.[26] The Sisters Study analyzed data collected from 586 women, some of whom had developed breast cancer, and their cancer-free siblings. As part of this research project, blood samples were taken for DNA analysis and information was collected from participants on their use of vitamins during the previous twelve years.

According to lead researcher Dr. Honglei Chen, head of the Aging and Neuroepidemiology Group at the U.S. National Institute of Environmental Health Sciences, it was discovered during the Sister Study that "multivitamin use was associated with longer leukocyte telomeres." Telomeres, the end portion of chromosomes, protect against damage, but shorten each time cells divide. It is generally believed that this process sets limits to the number of possible cell divisions and, as a result, to lifespan.[27] The Sister Study showed that telomeres were, on average, 5.1 percent longer in women that had taken multivitamins. This greater length corresponds to about 9.8 years less age-related telomere shortening. While this evidence is not conclusive, it is highly suggestive that taking multivitamin supplements increases life expectancy. This is not surprising. In their book *Feel Better, Live Longer with Vitamin B3*,[28] two of the current authors pointed out that doctors inducted into the Orthomolecular Hall of Fame so far had lived an average of eighty-three years. Again, this greater than normal lifespan is not conclusive but is highly suggestive, especially since many of these inductees were born in the nineteenth century when general life expectancy was lower than it is today.

While adverse side-effects are the hallmark of conventional drug-based medicine, they are exceptionally uncommon in the practice of orthomolecular treatments. Once the new paradigm is widely adopted, treatments will go into areas untouched by conventional medicine. Nutritional mixtures are already available that can mitigate serious surgical and genetic brain damage, significantly improve antisocial behavior, and enormously reduce the incidence of both infectious and chronic degenerative diseases. As will now be demonstrated, niacin will be highly involved in the coming orthomolecular revolution.

A GENETIC HYPOTHESIS TO ACCOUNT FOR THE NEED FOR VITAMIN B3 BY SO MANY

The synthesis of niacin from tryptophan is a very inefficient process, and 60 mg of the amino acid are necessary to provide 1 mg of niacin. This process also involves vitamins B_1, B_2 and B_6. It also requires vitamin C for the first reaction catalyzed by indoleamine 2,3-dioxygenase. If these vitamins are in short supply, the synthesis of vitamin B_3 will be even less efficient. It must also be remembered that tryptophan itself is not usually very readily available in diet, especially if that diet contains a high level of corn.

It is clear, therefore, that humans have the ability to synthesize niacin, but this process is ineffective and is probably in evolutionary decline. Of course, Vitamin B_3 is also available from many foods. If diet contained enough of this vitamin to supply bodily requirements, there would be no need to convert tryptophan to niacin. This would liberate energy for other uses and free up tryptophan for the production of serotonin, a major neurotransmitter. Humanity has been depending more and more on vitamin B_3 derived from diet, but recently niacin has become less available from food. As a result, subclinical pellagra and other niacin deficiency disorders are becoming very widespread.

According to Miller,[29] tuberculosis (TB) is one such example of niacin deficiency and a very important factor in the evolution of schizophrenia. In a very thorough study of the relationship between schizophrenia and tuberculosis. Miller formulated the reasonable hypothesis that the rapid spread of tuberculosis, which began with the dawn of industrialization, was due to the evolution of the bacteria so that it became more persistent in the human body and easily transferred to others.

Many years ago, a surgeon called me (AH) and told me that he had tuberculosis of the pericardium and that none of the drugs used had stopped the infection. He was so weak he could barely dress or look after himself, concentrate, or read. In my tuberculosis reprint file, I had several papers published many years ago showing that niacin inhibited the growth of the bacterium. I gave him the references and suggested that he take 1,000 mg niacin three times daily after meals along with the same amount of ascorbic acid (vitamin C). Two weeks later he called back. He was now able to concentrate and read, and had a lot more energy. A couple of years later, I suddenly remembered him and called him at his hospital. To my surprise, he was not able to come to the phone because he was busy in the operating room.

I sent this little case history to Miller, who replied, "What I envision is this—that in the TB-infected tissue, the bacterium is pumping out niacin by depleting NAD (nicotinamide adenine dinucleotide) and furthermore, must somehow inhibit the recycling of niacin into NAD by producing an inhibitor of the host NAPRT1 enzyme. However, dietary niacin (as you provided the TB patient) would allow their non-TB-infected tissue to generate NAD and thereby save the host from the huge NAD sink that TB represents. Obviously, low NAD in all tissues equals death."

Unless their diet is high in niacin or tryptophan, schizophrenics may still not have optimal NAD (though not anywhere close to the near-death levels in TB patients) because the deficiency of the niacin receptor causes a compensatory shift towards niacin conservation. The prediction is that these patients should be more resistant to TB than their ethnically matched counterparts, because the niacin receptor deficiency keeps the kynurenine pathway activated.

NAD is central to the model presented here for the intersection of two diseases, poised in the balance between disease susceptibility and disease resistance. The sheer magnitude of the importance of NAD to bioenergetic homeostasis provides the driving force for the compromise of related pathways. Thus, the architects of new pharmaceuticals for schizophrenia and for TB would do well to incorporate an in-depth understanding of the many nuances of the pathways to NAD.

There is a great deal of evidence to support this argument. Some 50 percent of the population of the developed world seems to suffer from disorders or diseases that respond beneficially to niacin or niacinamide supplementation. This figure is probably an underestimate. Sufferers from arthritis (20 percent), addictions (10 percent), children with learning and/or behavioral disorders (5 percent), cardiovascular disease, coronary disease and stroke (30 percent), cancer (50 percent), schizophrenia, or severe stress (unknown) would very likely improve if given more niacin.

This brings us back to diseases associated with niacin deficiency. Hoffer and Foster have shown there are numerous, extremely dangerous diseases and disorders associated with our inability to synthesize adequate vitamin B_3. Any genetic aberration promoting such a deficiency state, if it was to widely diffuse in the human population, must have carried with it some enormous counterbalancing advantage(s). If it did not, it would soon have disappeared from the human gene pool. What then are the advantages of the apparent inadequate synthesis of niacin?

Schizophrenic genes are good genes. Dr. David Horrobin[30] was convinced that the introduction of the schizophrenic genes into our genetic configuration was largely responsible for the creation of our modern society. Schizophrenic genes could not have survived millions of years of evolution unless they conferred some evolutionary advantage[31]—and they do—but only for the healthy relatives of patients. There is no advantage in being sick, and society usually treated these unfortunate patients so badly that they could not possibly have had any evolutionary advantage. If a person becomes schizophrenic at age forty-five and until then has been normally productive and creative, it surely means there is not much really wrong with their genes but that some long-term environmental trigger factors are responsible instead. It means that these genes, which have been normal for forty-five years, are no longer able to obtain the nutrients from their environment that they must have in order to remain well.

The Evolutionary Advantages of Having Schizophrenic Genes

Schizophrenic patients, before they become sick and after they recover, have many physical and psychological advantages over the population lacking these genes. Physically they are more attractive; they age more gracefully. Their hair does not gray as quickly. They can withstand severe pain better. They become arthritic less often and they have cancer much less frequently, and when they do get cancer they recover when treated by standard and orthomolecular methods. Out of over 5,000 schizophrenic patients and over 1,500 cancer cases that I (AH) have treated since 1955, only eleven had both diseases.[32] All but one recovered with orthomolecular treatment combined with standard treatment for their cancer.

Schizophrenic patients' first-order relatives also are protected against cancer but not to the same degree. I have seen many families with many cases of cancer and very few schizophrenics, and families with many schizophrenic members and hardly any cases of cancer. The following table records what I had observed.

	NUMBER OF RELATIVES	NUMBER WITH SCHIZOPHRENIA	NUMBER WITH CANCER	NUMBER OF INDEX CASES
Cancer	785	3	89	114
Schizophrenia	437	20	26	95

This natural antagonism between these two major diseases also applies to first-order families (parents, siblings, and children)—there is a striking difference in incidence.

The best explanation I have been able to come up with for this correlation is that both schizophrenia and cancer are adrenochrome diseases. One of the major causes of schizophrenia is too much adrenochrome, and one of the major causes of cancer is too little. Adrenochrome is a hallucinogen and also has antimitotic properties because it inhibits cell division, and cancer, of course, is cell division that has gone rampant. Since all the schizophrenic patients were treated with vitamin B_3 (niacin or niacinamide) and ascorbic acid, this suggests that the clear differences I observed were also related to these two vitamins. The conclusion is that schizophrenic patients on niacin and vitamin C will get cancer less frequently than either the same patients not on these vitamins or the nonschizophrenic population. Professor Diona Damian's finding that niacinamide protects the skin against UVA and UVB rays and was more effective than sunscreens in protecting against skin cancer and protects the immune function of the skin was reported by *The Sydney Morning Herald* in November 19, 2008. Perhaps it has the same effect in protecting against all cancers. Niacin will be as effective as niacinamide as they are interconvertible in the body. Niacin might be even be better, as it tends to increase pigmentation of the skin. This has led to the erroneous idea that niacin causes acanthosis nigricans, a skin disorder, which it does not (see Chapter 5).

> People with the schizophrenic good genes have an evolutionary advantage, but they have to be fed properly. They need vitamin B_3, and relief from excessive oxidation in the body. It is as if schizophrenic episodes use, deplete, and ultimately demand more vitamin B_3. This requirement must be met with supplementation as it cannot be met by the normal diet.

Psychologically, schizophrenics are more creative and enterprising than the nonschizophrenic population. They tend to see relationships in the world that the rest of us do not see. The psychedelic drug LSD experience has a similar effect. Many years ago we studied the psychedelic reaction as a way of enhancing creativity. Many brilliant writers, poets, artists, and even Nobel Laureates had these good genes.

Schizophrenia: The Clinical Picture

Schizophrenia is characterized by a combination of perceptual changes and thought disorder, which may lead to strange or psychotic behavior. When schizophrenic patients are well, however—either before they become sick or after they have recovered—they do posses several physical and psychological advantages. If schizophrenia is caused by hyperoxidation of the catecholamines, leading to increased production of adrenochrome and similar chrome indoles, then it should be possible to predict what the syndrome will be like as an intellectual exercise, simply by knowing the properties of adrenalin and adrenochrome.

Adrenochrome has the following properties, and each should lead to the described consequences in schizophrenic patients:

1. A neurotransmitter inhibitor: perceptual changes and thought disorder—True.
2. A mitotic inhibitor: interference with growth if first occurs in childhood; decreased incidence of cancer; better response of the cancer to treatment—True.
3. Toxic to heart muscle: increased incidence of cardiac disease—True.
4. Formation of melanin pigments: skin changes in pellagra and in some schizophrenic patients—True.
5. Patients made worse by oxidative stress—True.
6. Antioxidants are therapeutic—True

Schizophrenia can be triggered by factors, which increase oxidative stress. Conversely, antioxidants and decreased stress will be therapeutic. Schizophrenia is characterized by changes due to sensory misinterpretations of stimuli and an inability to judge that these changes are not true. Psychotic behavior is comprehensible if one determines the perceptual distortions.

Evolution and Niacin Dependency

Adrenochrome and similar compounds, in common with the hallucinogens, cause perceptual changes. Vitamin B_3 is required to prevent excessive oxidation of adrenalin to adrenochrome in the brain. Factors which facilitate formation of NAD from tryptophan and B_3 supplements will be therapeutic. Possessors of the "schizophrenic good genes" have an evolutionary advantage (more creative; less cancer) but they have to receive proper nutrition to counter the schizophrenia. They need vitamin B_3, and increased use of antioxidants to relieve oxidative conditions in the body.

Yes, there is an evolutionary advantage conferred by vitamin B_3-dependent genes. The energy needed to transform tryptophan to NAD becomes available for other uses. The increased oxidation to adrenochrome and similar oxidized catecholamines provides protection against cancer and arthritis and perhaps many more diseases except heart disease. The decreased prevalence of cancer in these patients and their families will lead to a spread of these genes into the total population given enough time. Ideally only a little adrenochrome would be made, as may be the case with first-order relatives. But whether a little or too much is made, the individual is protected by taking optimum amounts of vitamin B_3. This will protect against the effect of adrenochrome on the brain and will also protect the heart by keeping cholesterol levels normal. In time, due to evolutionary pressure, we will all have these schizophrenic genes but no one will be sick because we will be adding enough B_3 to our food to replace what our bodies no longer can make and need.

In 1960, Dr. Osmond and I (AH) suggested the following criteria for a good hypothesis. First: It must account both inclusively and economically for what is known already; a hypothesis that fails to do this would be automatically disqualified. Second: It must do this better than any previous hypothesis. Third: It must be testable in a way that will readily lead to its refutation should it be false, using methods available to science under scrutiny. It should also be useful in directing research into productive areas. Is there any reason why psychiatry should require anything different from the rest of science?

I think our adrenochrome hypothesis meets all these criteria. It does take into account most of the clinical findings in schizophrenic patients but of course can not account for the large number of biochemical findings that are being discovered. It takes into account clinical findings but cannot be compared to any previous hypothesis, as none have been as inclusive and comprehensive. The purely psychological hypotheses of schizophrenia have been dismal failures and have hurt many patients and their families. Biochemical hypotheses have been crude and have not led anywhere. Infection hypotheses may play a minor role, as any serious brain pathology can produce the schizophrenic syndrome. The adrenochrome hypothesis is testable and has been tested to a limited degree but unfortunately, psychiatry has been too preoccupied with drugs and the minutia of how they work to look comprehensively in this direction. It has finally led to the treatment of schizophrenia using orthomolecular methods, which are much more successful than using only drugs. Thousands of schizophrenic patients became normal on orthomolecular therapy.

DEFICIENCY AND DEPENDENCY

A deficiency is present when the amount of any nutrient in the diet is below what the average person needs. Classically it applies to the well-known deficiency diseases such as scurvy, beriberi, pellagra, and rickets. Scurvy is caused by deficiency of ascorbic acid. This deficiency alone has killed millions of people. Pellagra is caused by too little vitamin B_3 in the diet. Supplementation with these vitamins prevented these diseases. This was the basis of the old vitamins-as-prevention paradigm developed about 100 years ago and reluctantly accepted by the medical profession about 50 years ago. Since then it has become so solidly established, it is as if it is written in stone, even though it is totally out of date, wrong, and harmful to so many patients. It is inadequate because it assumes that every one has the same nutritional needs. That is like assuming that everyone has the same fingerprints. A large number of people have much higher vitamin requirements than our modern diets can provide, and if they depend upon their diet alone, they will never achieve optimum health. For these people, the correct term is dependency.

A deficiency will become a dependency if the deficiency is chronic. The rapidity with which this occurs depends on several factors including severity of the stress, severity of the malnutrition, and iatrogenic (physician-induced) causes. These are trigger factors. The European concentration camps and prisoner of war camps in the Far East were ideal for throwing people into the dependency state if they lived long enough. In the Japanese war camps, Canadian soldiers were incarcerated for forty-four months. There they suffered severe malnutrition from a diet of about 800 calories daily, which caused several deficiency diseases. This was combined with severe physical and psychological stress. One-quarter of the prisoners died in camp. The remaining soldiers remained sick for the rest of their lives with the exception of a few who were given niacin, three grams daily, after their release.

The risk of becoming dependent varies with the duration and intensity of malnutrition, with the presence of disease such as infection of the gastrointestinal tract, food allergies, the duration and intensity of systemic infections, and with the level and duration of stress. When all three factors are operating at high levels, the time needed to become dependent will be shortened. Cleave[33] found that it took twenty years before saccharine disease developed on a high sugar, highly refined carbohydrate, and low-fiber diet without abnormal stress. The Canadian soldiers in Hong Kong camps became dependent in four years. But their malnutrition, presence of disease, and stress were much more severe.

Miller[34] suggests that tuberculosis increased susceptibility toward schizophrenia and that this has been a major factor in driving the evolutionary development of this disease. This bacterium depletes the body of its NAD by forcing an increased production of niacin, which is made from NAD. This ensures the survival of this infectious disease and its ready spread. It is uncommon in developed countries but is still a major pandemic in Africa, associated with the HIV virus. Tuberculosis is a trigger factor which converts a deficiency into a dependency.

Vitamin B_3-deficient and -dependent patients will share many symptoms but they will not be identical since the reason for the relative deficiency is different. The vitamin-deficient person is also lacking many other nutrients because their diet is so poor in quality. But the vitamin dependents may be dependent on only one vitamin and may be getting enough of the others from their diet.

Causes of the Dependency

The causes of B_3 dependency have not been studied because the concept has not been examined seriously. No doubt there are many reasons. The cause may be genetic and present from birth due to the absence of genes or the presence of defective enzymes. In the majority of cases they start to work after birth and may develop at an early age, but they also may come on toward the end of one's life. There are two major factors. One is that a long-term deficiency will become a dependency if the condition is not treated. The pellagrologists in the 1930s observed that when dealing with well-recognized cases of pellagra, there were a few who did not become well until the amount of B_3 was increased to 1,000 milligrams daily, although most would recover on very much less. They could not understand the reason for this. It was also shown that the canine equivalent of pellagra, called black tongue, showed the same variable responses. If dogs were maintained on a diet deficient in B_3 for a few months and then given the vitamin again, they would quickly recover on the usual small doses.

But if the dogs were deprived for more than six months, they would need much larger doses to recover. Being kept deficient eventually made these animals dependent. The same occurred with pellagra patients.

I think the same thing is happening today on a much wider scale. People who appear to be well for many years on a diet only mildly deficient will eventually become dependent. This accounts for the fact that so many of the modern diseases of our affluent society develop in middle age and later, although there is evidence that these conditions are beginning to appear much earlier than they used to. For example, if patients with early-onset arthritis with very little joint degradation but with pain and stiffness are given B$_3$, they recover very quickly. My (AH) mother, who at age sixty-six was developing typical arthritis with Heberden's nodes, was well after only one month on niacin, 1 gram three times daily after meals. She lived another twenty years and wrote two books during that time.

If the condition is allowed to damage the person for a long time, it will take much more vitamin and a much longer period of time to recover. The time required on a deficiency diet to convert into dependency depends upon the degree of deficiency. If it is mild it will take much longer. If it is severe, as it was in Japanese war camps, it will take only a few years. I think that with the average North American diet it may take twenty years. If the nutrients are replaced at any time during the development phase, the process can be interrupted; if the deficiency is slight, small amounts of vitamins will cure. These are found in the standard B-complex preparations, which contain almost all of the B-complex vitamins. If the deficiency has been prolonged and severe, taking multiple-vitamin preparations in the usual small doses will be of little help in counteracting the dependency. It would be like giving too little antibiotic for a disease when a large dose is needed. This will be disappointing to many who have heard from their friends how well they became on the small dose preparations, because they did not know their own needs were so much greater.

The second major cause is prolonged stress of any type, including malnutrition, chronic disease, and psychosocial stress including war and brutality. Post-traumatic stress disorder (PTSD) is a very common diagnosis. An example of severe stress was the experience of the above-mentioned Canadian soldiers in World War II, when they were incarcerated in Japanese prison camps for forty-four months. Other examples were the Holocaust camps, which killed most of the unfortunate prisoners. A current example is the enormous stress of unrest, malnutrition and starvation, disease, and war in Africa. These victims suffer from a combination of all three forms of stress. The adverse impacts of combined psychosocial stress, starvation, and malnutrition peaked in the concentration camps of Europe and the prisoner of war camps in the Far East.

Niacin and Prisoners of War

Here is how Hoffer and Foster have previously described the impact of severe niacin deprivation:

> The effects of this stress-malnutrition combination did not end upon release. Its subsequent impacts were obvious on the aging process. Over two thousand untrained Canadian soldiers were sent to Hong Kong to defend it from invasion from the east. But the Japanese attacked from the west and soon all these Canadian soldiers were in prison camps. Forty-four months later, one-quarter of them had died and the rest were left permanently impaired. On their way home in hospital ships, they were fed the strongest vitamin preparation then available, rice bran extracts, and apparently they rapidly began to regain their health. Those that had survived had lost up to one-third of their body weight [and now] began to replace some of this loss. Although they appeared to become well again, they did not. A survey conducted by the federal government established that they were much sicker than Canadian soldiers who had fought in Europe, and, as a result, they were given special pensions. After the war, they suffered to an exaggerated degree from all the diseases of aging, including arthritis, blindness, heart disease, neurological deterioration, and depression. Dr. Hoffer estimated that one year in a Far Eastern prisoner of war camp aged these soldiers about five years, as compared to a normal year living at home. A soldier imprisoned in such a camp at chronological age thirty-five would come out four years later with a biological age of fifty-five.
>
> One of these former Hong Kong veterans, GP, was the administrator of a retirement home for many elderly men and women. GP had been depressed, experienced severe arthritis, was fearful, was heat and cold intolerant and had spent some time on a psychiatric ward for veterans. He had been diagnosed as having a personality disorder. Much to his surprise after two weeks on niacin he became normal. All these

symptoms had disappeared and he remained well until he died years later as Lieutenant Governor for the Province of Saskatchewan. Through his intercession, some 20 more Hong Kong veterans as they were called and USA former prisoners of war came to see Dr. Hoffer. Given niacin treatment, they all recovered. It was concluded that the high dose niacin had reversed the health deterioration caused by the extraordinarily severe stress of these camps.[35]

Life was hell for these men. They were treated with extreme brutality, were starved of calories, vitamins, and minerals, and they suffered from many deficiency diseases including scurvy, pellagra, beriberi, and infections.

Hans Selye tried to develop a measure for the severity of stress. He defined severe stress as a set of circumstances that would kill 10 percent of the exposed animals. As these prisoners died at a rate two and a half times greater than that, clearly mankind has been exposed to terrible stress indeed. When the soldiers were freed shortly after the atomic bomb was dropped, the doctors in charge knew what was wrong. The men were fed the crude vitamin preparations then available on the hospital ships that brought them back to Victoria (see quotation above). These soldiers appeared to recover, but in fact they had not. Their subsequent loss due to disability and death has been enormous, yet little attention was given to the plight of these veterans.

In response to continuous complaints from the Hong Kong Veterans Association, Dr. Richardson (1964–1965) compared the health of a sample of these veterans against their brothers who had served in Europe. The Hong Kong veterans were as a group much sicker. The death rate from heart disease was greater, and the incidence of crippling arthritis, nervousness, tension, weakness, blindness, and depression was much higher. In recognition of these findings, Hong Kong veterans receive higher pensions. It became clear that these men have been deteriorating both physically and mentally at a rate much higher than normal, and higher than that of soldiers who were not exposed to severe stress and malnutrition. William Allister was one of the Canadians held in these camps. He died at eighty-nine. His obituary describes the severe stress they suffered.[36]

The history of one small sample of veterans (around twelve), is much different, for they have been taking 3 grams of niacin per day. These twelve recovered and remained well as long as they took this quantity of vitamin regularly. One of the last three survivors in Victoria died on July 2006. He was over eighty years old and had been on niacin for several decades and getting on well. He died of a coronary heart attack, but his last few weeks were marred by the hospital not allowing him to stay on his niacin. He felt terrible over this, as did his wife. This is another example of cruelty to patients for absolutely no reason whatever aside from rigid nutritional ignorance.

One of these survivors was Mr. GP, who was sick from the time he came back to Canada in 1944. His Veterans Administration file—all five pounds of it—got thicker, but he did not get any better. Most of the file contained results of frequent medical examinations and investigations. Throughout this period, GP was heavily medicated with amphetamines to keep him alert during the day and barbiturates to allow him to sleep at night. He did not get well on this regime. On one occasion he was investigated in a psychiatric ward, which made him worse.

GP suffered from arthritis so incapacitating that he and his wife had to work up to one hour each morning to mobilize him so he could go to work. He also suffered from chronic anxiety and fear for which he received psychotherapy. For example, he would not sit in any room with his back to the door. On his way to Hong Kong he was a healthy young physical instructor about six feet tall, weighing around 190 pounds. When he came back to Canada, his weight was around 120 pounds. Even though he regained his weight and apparently was well, this was not really the case. Eventually he was treated in a Veterans Administration hospital, where he was diagnosed as suffering from anxiety. In fact he was suffering because he could not function properly.

In 1960 I started a project to study the effect of niacin on aging patients. GP was the director of the institution housing the patients, so I described the effects of niacin, its flush, and so on to him. A few months later he asked me whether he could also take the vitamin. I wondered why he would want to, and he told me that it would be easier for him to explain the flush to the elderly men living there if he experienced it. At that time I knew nothing about his wartime background.

A few months later he told me that he was okay—and I did not know what he meant. Then he told me about his forty-four months in the prisoner of war camp. Two weeks after starting the niacin, his arthritis was gone, he was able to lift both arms high over his shoulders, he was no longer heat and cold intolerant, and he was no longer anxious. He suffered a relapse several years later when he forgot to take his niacin on a trip to the mountains with his son. Two weeks later he was well into a relapse, and he never forgot again. A medical health officer who had been in the same camp with GP could not believe that the niacin had been of any value and accused GP of having had a placebo response. Later GP—George Porteous is his real name—became Lieutenant Governor of Saskatchewan. He was very proud of his recovery and told as many people as would listen to him about it. And because he described his recovery so freely, he helped many Hong Kong Veterans and United States ex–POWs.

The Deficiency Dependency Continuum: From Pellagra to Schizophrenia

Vitamin B$_3$ deficiency produces a large variety of psychiatric syndromes. Green and Kaufman, independently, described this so well.[37,38,39] It appears that a good deal of modern psychiatry depends on patients suffering from unidentified pellagra for its bread and butter. They would do a much better job if the basic treatment restored the insufficient vitamin. At the extreme end of the optimum-need continuum, the syndrome is much more likely to be even more severe and chronic. This includes the psychoses of aging, bipolar disease, and schizophrenic psychoses. Therefore it is logical to drop the word "schizophrenia," and to use the correct term, pellagra, which would be described as light to severe or as brief or prolonged. The pellagra caused by a deficient diet could be called deficiency pellagra and the pellagra caused by an increased requirement would be called dependency pellagra.

Clinically, schizophrenia and the pellagra psychosis could not be distinguished from each other in the southern mental hospitals, where they had the most experience in dealing with these syndromes. The differential was made on the basis of what the patients ate and the typical skin color of the condition. When niacin became available as a treatment it was used—and the schizophrenic patients who recovered with small doses of niacin were rediagnosed as pellagra sufferers, while the schizophrenic patients who did not recover on the small dose continued to be diagnosed as schizophrenic. Schizophrenics did not have the same degree of skin discoloration because they were not exposed to the sun as much as the pellagrins.

The major clinical analysis accepted by the pellagrologists was that only pellagrins would respond to better diets and small amounts of niacin. They did try up to 1,000 milligrams daily and were surprised that a few pellagrins needed these higher doses, which was considered enormous in those days.

Since schizophrenia and the pellagra psychosis are almost identical, and since the differences can be readily accounted for by the fact that they represent extreme ends of the B_3-requirement continuum, why do we not use the correct name? The development of a dependency is related to the severity of the initial deficiency and its duration. People with a minor deficiency will present symptoms for a brief periods of time, say months rather than years, and will respond more quickly to smaller doses of the vitamin. They are like the pellagrins who responded so quickly to "vitamin" (small) doses of B_3, and like the dogs with black tongue that were not kept deficient too long. Schizophrenic patients have been on a deficient diet for years rather than months and they need large doses of B_3. They will also respond more slowly to treatment, as did the chronic pellagrins and the black tongue dogs that were maintained on a deficient diet too long.

In "High-affinity Niacin Receptor HM74A is Decreased in the Anterior Cingulate," Miller and Dulay's last paragraph states:

> In conclusion, one important implication of the data we present here is that the early clinical studies by Abram Hoffer reported in a notable degree of success through treatment of unmedicated patients with niacin, but inconsistently replicated in follow-up work by others, should now be re-evaluated in the context of the limitation imposed by a deficient receptor, . . . The possibility that a deficiency in the high-affinity receptor is a core feature of many individuals with schizophrenia provides a basis for research into more potent receptor agonists and therapies that might significantly increase expression of the fully-functional protein.[40]

Miller and Dulay's research provides us for the first time with a clear indication what is one of the causes of schizophrenia. The nicotinic acid receptors are not functioning properly, either because there are too few, or because they are malformed, or because they are less responsive to the presence of this vitamin in the fluid external to the cells. Using the lock and key analogy, either the lock or the key are not right for each other, or there are too few pathways into the cell. This can be overcome by increasing the head of pressure into the cell by using large doses.

If it quacks like a duck, walks like a duck, looks like a duck, and flies like a duck, then surely it must be a duck. Pellagra is that duck.

Schizophrenia and pellagra are clinically the same, and often one cannot be distinguished from the other unless the niacin therapeutic test is given. They are both nutritional diseases with major social and economic implications, and they both respond to proper treatment with optimum doses of niacin. Pellagra is a B_3 deficiency condition: there is not enough in food to meet the patient's requirements. Pellagra is also a dependency disease because there is not enough niacin in even the best of diets, and it must be supplemented. The word *schizophrenia* is therefore redundant. Even more, it is damaging to patients, to their families, and to society. The correct word should be *pellagra,* which can be qualified by the term *dependency pellagra* to distinguish it from deficiency pellagra. Deficiency pellagra is, of course, also complicated by deficiencies of other vitamins, protein, and essential fatty acids. I hope Cato the Elder will not mind: *Schizophrenia delenda est.* (Schizophrenia must be eliminated.)

CHAPTER 4

How to Take Niacin

There is a principle which is a bar against all information,
which is proof against all argument, and which cannot fail
to keep man in everlasting ignorance. That principle
is condemnation without investigation.
—WILLIAM PALEY (1743–1805),
OFTEN ATTRIBUTED TO HERBERT SPENCER (1820–1903)

The keys to taking niacin therapy are *quantity*, *frequency*, and *duration*. You need to take enough, take it frequently, and take it long enough to see benefit.

TAKE ENOUGH

Adequately high supplement doses need to be employed to get the job done. As there is a certain, large amount of fuel needed to launch an aircraft or a spacecraft, there is a certain, large amount of a nutrient needed to cure a sick body. With vitamin therapy, speed of recovery is proportional to dosage used. Dr. Hoffer's standard prescription was 3,000 milligrams (mg) per day.

Much less is needed for prevention and daily good health maintenance. The Recommended Dietary Allowance (RDA) for niacin is under 18 mg per day. That is far too low. In 2007, an independent review panel of twenty-two researchers and physicians issued their recommendation for niacin intake for an adult: 300 mg per day.[1]

TAKE FREQUENTLY

Niacin is a water-soluble vitamin. This means that it is lost from the body easily during the course of a day or even a few hours. Therefore, divide the daily niacin dose and take a third of it with every meal. Taking niacin with meals improves absorption.

Dr. William Kaufman and other experienced physicians have advocated for the importance of the frequency of doses. With the water-soluble vitamins, at any given quantity, frequently-divided doses are invariably more effective. (There is more about Dr. Kaufman's treatment for arthritis in Chapter 7.)

TAKE IT LONG ENOUGH

Some persons will notice benefits right away. Blood lipid benefits take more time. Long-standing mental illness may respond slowly, over a period of weeks or even months. Every patient is different, and this is why we recommend that you work in close cooperation with your personal physician.

HOW DO I KNOW IF NIACIN IS HELPING?

There are two ways to tell if your niacin supplementation is working for you: subjectively and objectively.

Subjective Proof

If you are fighting mental illness, you will know full well when you feel better. It is just that simple. Friends and family may comment positively. Dr. Hoffer's standard measure of recovery was this: recovered, truly well patients pay income tax. It sounds odd, but a person must be successfully holding a job in order to do so. Placebos rarely achieve that result. Critics of Hoffer's work have claimed that it was his pleasant, positive bedside manner that resulted in cured patients. Dr. Hoffer replied, "I am nice to all my patients. However, only the ones getting niacin get better."

> **Common sense caution:** Work with your doctor. Persons with a history of heavy alcohol use, liver disorders, diabetes, or pregnancy will especially want to have their physician monitor their use of niacin in quantity.

Objective Proof

Ask your physician to check and see. For example, laboratory tests can easily verify if your blood lipids are benefiting from niacin. Watch especially for lower triglycerides, and higher "good" HDL.

HOW MUCH IS TOO MUCH?

A person's absolute upper limit for niacin is the amount that causes nausea, and, if not reduced, vomiting. The dose should never be allowed to remain at this upper limit. Dr. Hoffer's usual therapeutic dose range was 3,000 mg daily, divided into three doses of 1,000 mg each. Sometimes some patients need more. The toxic dose for dogs is about 5,000 mg per 2.2 pounds (1 kilogram) of body weight. We do not know the toxic dose for humans since niacin has never killed anyone.

We think that monitoring long-term use of niacin is a good idea for anyone. It consists of having your doctor periodically (perhaps once or twice a year) check your liver function with a simple blood test. Correct interpretation of these monitoring tests is important.

Niacin is not liver toxic, but niacin therapy does increase liver function tests. This elevation means that the liver is active—it does not indicate an underlying liver pathology.

So-Called "Safe Upper Limits"

In spite of all this, there is now a government-sponsored "Safe Upper Limit" (or "tolerable upper intake level") for niacin consumption. It is 35 mg per day.[2] We offer this book as a charge-leading rebuttal against the arbitrariness and absurdity of that figure. Among many reasons why it is preposterous is that the so-called Safe Upper Limit is only about twice the RDA! There is no clinical or laboratory evidence whatsoever that proves that niacin, or any other vitamin, is dangerous at double the RDA.

Instead, authoritative-sounding speculation is offered to the public in the form of statements like this: "Supplement users at risk from ignorance of tolerable upper limits . . . Consuming too many nutrients can lead to harmful side-effects, a fact many users were worryingly unaware of, said researchers . . . (T)he tolerable upper level of one B vitamin, niacin, was exceeded by nearly 50 per cent of all the participants in their study who reported taking supplements . . . (D)ietary supplements exceeding the tolerable upper limits were fairly common in the U.S., as the supplement industry is not regulated in the same way as pharmaceutical industry."[3]

The authors of this paper claim that side-effect symptoms will likely occur in half of those persons taking 100 mg of supplemental niacin, and that it is impossible to identify those who are at greatest risk.[4] We consider such statements to be scaremongering and sensationalism.

In his fifty-five years of experience with thousands of patients, Dr. Hoffer found that even 40,000 mg of niacin daily is not toxic. He estimated that over 200,000 mg per day is fatal. There is a built in safety valve with niacin: vomiting. Nausea will occur far in advance of any risk of fatality. Most of us would never exceed a few thousand mg daily, an amount that orthodox physicians frequently give patients to raise HDL. The safety margin is very large. For more than twenty-five years, data collected by the American Association of Poison Control Centers (AAPCC) confirms that there is not even one niacin-related death per year. (Download any Annual Report of the American Association of Poison Control Centers from 1983–2009 free of charge at http://www.aapcc.org/. The "Vitamin" category is usually near the end of the report.)

THE NIACIN FLUSH AND VASODILATATION (VASODILATION)

Niacin usually causes a flush a few minutes after it is taken. A few people will flush with 25 mg, more with 50 mg, and most with 100 mg. The flush begins in the forehead and works its way down the body, rarely affecting

Vitamins: How Much to Take?

In his classic health book, *Supernutrition*,[5] Richard A. Passwater suggests a simple and utterly nontechnical method to determine what amounts of vitamins you personally need to take for optimum health. Wisely, no one prescriptive list is given; no "one size fits all" approach is offered. Rather, Dr. Passwater builds a careful and well-documented case for megavitamin therapy, and then shows how to increase your own vitamin doses in two-week intervals until peak health has been achieved. Essentially, you take the smallest amounts of supplements that give the greatest results. If you go over and beyond that level, your health benefits will stay the same or decline. That would be the point of diminishing returns, the point of wasting money, and/or a potentially harmful overdose. If this seems like common sense, perhaps that's because it is. Interestingly, when doctors use this very same approach with drugs, it is called a "therapeutic trial." With drugs, it is trial and error. With nutrients, it is trial and much, much less risk of error.

the toes. The higher the initial dose the greater the initial flush, but if any dose causes a maximum flush a larger dose taken later will not cause a greater flush. The capillaries are dilated and the blood flow through the organs is increased. There is an internal increase in blood flow as well as in the skin, which may last up to several hours. Patients must be warned that this will happen. If not, they may be very surprised and even shocked. Patients can be started on lower doses until they have adjusted to the decreased intensity of the flush. Then the doses may be increased gradually.

> With large initial doses, the niacin flush is more pronounced and lasts longer. But with each additional dose, the intensity of the flush decreases and in most patients becomes a minor nuisance rather than an irritant. To minimize flushing, niacin should always be taken right after finishing one's meal.

Each time the niacin is taken, the flush is repeated but to a much lesser degree. In most cases it is almost all gone after a week or so, and is a minor nuisance at worst. However, some patients do not tolerate the flush and will have to discontinue the niacin. Non-flush preparations are available for these subjects (see Chapter 1). If the routine is interrupted for several days and then resumed, the same sequence of flushing will occur, but the initial flush usually will not be as strong as the original one. The intensity of the flush is minimized by taking the pills after meals and by taking them regularly, three times daily. I (AH) have been taking niacin for fifty-five years and at most have very minor flushes. It is a drier flush, not like the wet menopausal flush, or the flush suffered by male hormone blockers used in treating prostate cancer. Niacinamide does not cause flushing in the majority of patients. In perhaps 1 percent of patients, it will cause a very unpleasant flush, in which case it cannot be used. Probably their bodies convert the niacinamide into niacin too rapidly. This is unlikely to be you.

Vasodilatation (often called vasodilation) is sometimes very helpful. Many patients, particularly arthritics, have reported that they feel much better when their joints are warmed up by the flush and some will stop taking niacin for a few days in order to experience the flush once more. But for most patients, the sensation is not pleasant. It is tolerable if patients know what to expect and are properly prepared by the physician. William Parsons Jr. writes that only physicians who know niacin should use it. No-flush and slow-release preparations, which are also no-flush, are available. The best known no-flush product is inositol hexaniacinate, which is an ester of inositol, a vitamin, and niacin. I have used it with success for many years and consider it less effective compared to niacin. Doubling the niacin dose may be needed. But only trial and error will determine which is best for some patients.

Some Histamine History

Back in 1962, with only about a decade of niacin research behind me, I (AH) wrote: "Little is known about the physiology of the nicotinic acid vasodilatation; it resembles histamine flushing in its mode of onset, unpleasantness, and bodily distribution but in contrast to the histamine-induced flush, there is no fall in blood pressure. Possibly it releases a histamine-like substance, either histamine itself or serotonin." Edmond Boyle, then director of research at the Miami Heart Institute, believed the dilatation was caused by the histamine released. He had examined the mast cells [found in skin and connective tissue, and the mucous linings of the nose, mouth, lungs, and digestive tract] before and after taking niacin and had seen that the mast cell vesicles containing histamine were empty after the flush. It is believed that niacin causes a flush by a complicated mechanism which releases histamine, interferes in prostaglandin metabolism, may be related to serotonin mechanism, and may involve the cholinergic system.[6]

Histamine is clearly involved. The typical niacin flush is identical with the flush produced by an injection of histamine. It is dampened down, if not prevented entirely, by antihistamines and by some of the original tranquilizers such as chlorpromazine. The adaptation to niacin is readily explained by the reduction in histamine in the storage sites such as the mast cells. When these are examined after a dose of histamine, these cells contain empty vesicles which contained the histamine and also heparinoids. If the next dose is spaced closely enough, there will have been no time for the storage sites to be refilled, and therefore less histamine will be available to be released. After there is complete adaptation to niacin, a rest of several days will start the flushing cycle again. This decrease in histamine has some advantage in reducing the effects of rapidly released histamine. Dr. Edmond Boyle found that guinea pigs treated with niacin were not harmed by anaphylactic shock. Because the flush is relatively transient, it can not be involved in the lowering of cholesterol, which remains in effect as long as niacin is continued. Prostaglandins appear to be involved. Thus, aspirin[7] and indomethacin[8] reduce the intensity of the flush[9].

Boyle found that niacin increased basophil leukocyte count. These white blood cells store histamine and heparin, and protect the body against microorganisms causing disease. We earlier implicated a histamine-glycosaminoglycan histaminase system as well as histamine in lipid absorption and redistribution. Boyle suggested that the improvement caused by niacin is much greater than can be explained by its effect on cholesterol. He thought it might be due to the release of histamine and to the eventual reduction in the intravascular "sludging" of blood cells."[10] Cheng et al. presented evidence that prostaglandins are involved in the niacin flush but they admit "the flushing is not completely understood."[11] I am sorry the histamine idea was shelved, as I think there is powerful evidence that it too is involved in the flushing process. Probably all these systems are interrelated.

When histamine is injected subcutaneously (under the skin) there is almost an immediate flush, which is indistinguishable from the niacin flush in distribution and intensity. However, when niacin is taken along with histamine, the flush is not immediate. It may come on much more slowly unless histamine is injected intravenously, in which case the flush is immediate. The flush that occurs following injection of niacin alone is identical to the flush observed when histamine is injected subcutaneously. The niacin flush, however, typically is not associated with a decrease in blood pressure as it is with the histamine flush.

Factors in Flushing

The rapidity with which the flush appears depends upon the concentration of niacin achieved. When taken by mouth with a meal or snack, the rate of absorption largely depends on the amount of food in the stomach: more food means slower absorption and less flushing. Another variable would be taking niacin with either a hot or cold beverage: more flushing is likely with a hot drink. Medication is another factor. Look up any prescription or over-the-counter drug that you are taking in the *Physicians' Desk Reference* or any of the many online drug facts/side effects/interactions websites. If the niacin is absorbed rapidly, the flush will come on more quickly. Lower doses induce the flush after a time period that varies enormously from person to person. The flush also depends on unknown resistance factors. A few cannot tolerate even a small dose of niacin, say fifty mg, before they flush, and have such severe flushes that they can not take any niacin except no-flush preparations (discussed in Chapter 1). A very few cannot even tolerate the no-flush preparations. Their histamine storage sites may be too sensitive and release histamine too quickly. Oddly enough, the best "no-flush preparation" is uninterrupted use of niacin. The flush returns if the niacin is not taken for a day or more, but when it is resumed, the original flush is not as intense.

Schizophrenic patients are usually less disturbed by the flush. Many schizophrenic patients do not flush until after several months and for as long as up to several years after starting to take 3 grams of niacin daily. This inability to flush may be related to their disease, for an appreciable number of schizophrenic patients begin to flush after several years of medication. This is a good prognostic sign and usually coincides with complete recovery. When I was treating schizophrenic patients with injections of histamine, I increased the dose until their diastolic pressure decreased to zero while they were lying on the bed. Patients remained comfortable throughout. Also, elderly patients and, oddly, children do not flush as heavily as adults.

These observations suggest that there may be a two-phase process occurring. The first involves the prostaglandins, which become activated and stimulate the release of histamine. If the prostaglandin reaction is primary, this would explain why the time to flush is variable, as it would depend upon the amount of histamine released. If the histamine release came first, the flush should be almost immediate. The way to test this hypothesis would be to check histamine blood levels as a kind of histamine tolerance test. I would expect that after niacin, there would not be an immediate release with little histamine in the blood, and later it would build up in concordance with the intensity of the flush. This two-phase reaction would account for the anti-flush effect of some of the antihistamines and the older antipsychotic drugs, which act on the histamine system. It would also explain the effect of aspirin, which acts on the prostaglandin system. (By the way, Kunin, who was the first to observe that aspirin is a partial antidote to the niacin flush, is hardly ever given any credit.)

Niacin Reduces Anaphylactic Shock

While he was working at Henry Wellcome Laboratories, Nobel Laureate Sir

Henry Dale discovered that histamine was released during anaphylaxis, a life-threatening allergic reaction. This is a very complex, severe reaction, and apparently acetyl choline and heparin are also involved. Guinea pigs are very sensitive to anaphylactic shock. Boyle found that if guinea pigs were pretreated for a week with niacin, they did not die after a second dose of protein—a procedure that killed all the animals not pretreated.

Common sense caution: Anaphylactic shock is life threatening. Work closely with your doctor if you have any history of this or other severe reactions. It is generally safe for your doctor to try a supervised therapeutic trial of niacin. It is unwise for you to do it alone.

I have used this technique to protect patients against anaphylactic shock. In 1996 I saw a man who was very fearful for his life. He was peanut sensitive and avoided all traces of peanuts, but over a six-month period he had five major reactions and nearly died from the last one. I advised him to start with ascorbic acid, 1 gram taken after each of three meals. Ascorbic acid destroys histamine, which is why scorbutic patients who are deficient in this vitamin have high blood histamine levels. I wanted to build up his blood ascorbic acid levels. After one week he was to take 100 mg of niacin three times daily after meals. This was designed to release a small amount of histamine with a gentle flush. My hypothesis was that the histamine would be destroyed by the ascorbic acid and would therefore be neutralized to a degree. The niacin dose was increased to 250 mg twice a day. This was his maintenance dose. He came back ten years later for an unrelated problem. He had not taken any niacin the previous two years after his doctor told him to stop. (This is an example of a totally illogical fear of niacin when the same doctor would, with no hesitation, prescribe any and all of the toxic drugs that are available.) I advised him to resume the niacin and to increase the dose until he was on 1 gram after each of three meals. He had no more reactions. I had advised him to be as careful as before.

I have also used the combination of niacin and ascorbic acid to protect patients against the hives induced by insect bites. And I found it very helpful in decreasing the intensity of the allergic reactions, no matter what type of substance the patient is reacting to, although it will not completely prevent these reactions.

Other Clinical Uses of Niacin

Some additional and interesting therapeutic uses of niacin include treatment of Meniere's syndrome (ringing in the ears plus nausea) and high-tone deafness. In long-term therapy, improvement was obtained with only 150–250 mg daily.[12] Resistance to x-radiation was greatly improved at around 500–600 mg daily. Radiation-induced nausea was also reduced. Supplemental niacin could therefore be of great value for cancer patients undergoing radiation therapy. Even healing after surgical shock and other trauma including burns, hemorrhage, and infection is more rapid with niacin administration. More clinical uses of niacin are discussed in Chapter 11.

To Flush or Not to Flush? The Niacin Flush as Dosage Indicator

I (AWS)have found that the best way to accurately control the flushing sensation is to start with small amounts of niacin and gradually increase the dosage until the first flush is noticed. If you are new to all of this, one very gentle method is to start with a mere 25 mg three times a day, most likely with each meal. The next day, try 50 mg at breakfast, 25 mg at lunch, and 25 mg at supper. The following day, increase the dose to 50 mg at breakfast, 50 mg at lunch, and 25 mg at supper, and the next day take 50 mg at each of the three meals. Continue increasing the dosage by taking 75 mg, 50 mg, and 50 mg the next day, then 75 mg, 75 mg, and 50 mg, and so on. In this way you have increased at the easy rate of only 25 mg per day. You would continue to increase the dosage by 25 mg per day until the flush occurs.

It may take quite a while. It is difficult to predict your personal optimum level for niacin because each person is different. As a general rule, the more you can hold without flushing, the more you need. If you flush early, you don't need much niacin. If flushing doesn't happen until a high level, then your body is utilizing (and needs) the higher amount of the vitamin.

Now that you've had your first flush, what's next? Since a flush often indicates temporary saturation of niacin, it is desirable to continue to repeat the flushing, just very slightly, to continue the saturation. This could be done three or more times a day. Niacin can be taken to saturation at bedtime too, to get to sleep sooner at night. You might be asleep before you even notice the flush.

An important point here is that niacin is a vitamin, not a drug. It may relax you (a good thing) but it does not "put you to sleep" or anything like it. Niacin is not a hypnotic (sleeping pill). It is not habit forming. Niacin does not require a prescription because it is that safe. It is a nutrient that everyone needs each day. Different people in different circumstances require different amounts of niacin.

People in fairly good health often choose to increase their doses gradually in order to minimize flushing. If they do increase the dose slowly, what I describe is pretty accurate. For instance, I have been taking niacin for many years, in daily but varying doses depending on my stress level or dietary intake. I know by the flush when I've had enough for the moment. It is like turning off the hot water when the tub is full enough for a nice bath.

When you flush, you can literally see and feel that you've taken enough niacin, at least for now. The idea is to initially take just enough niacin to have a slight flush. This means a pinkness about the cheeks, ears, neck, forearms, and perhaps elsewhere. A slight niacin flush should end in about ten minutes or so. If you take too much niacin, the flush may be more pronounced and longer lasting. If you flush beet red for an hour, well, you took too much. Large doses of niacin on an empty stomach are certain to cause profound flushing.

Most people flush when they start niacin supplementation and gradually get adapted to it unless they stop for a few days and then resume. A few never get used to it, and they take the no-flush preparations. But the intensity of the flush is very variable. *Generally, people who need niacin the most flush the least.* That includes arthritics, schizophrenics, and people with cardiovascular problems. Some schizophrenics do not flush until they get well and *then* they begin to flush. *But the presence of the flush or its intensity cannot be uniquely used to measure the need for niacin,* as there are too many variables such as food in the stomach, whether the drink taken with it is hot or cold, the kind of food taken with it, and other medications the patient takes. Antipsychotics reduce the intensity of the flush as do aspirin and antihistamines.

Plain niacin may be purchased in tablets at many pharmacies, discount stores, health food stores, or online. Tablets typically are available in 50 mg, 100 mg, 250 mg, or 500 mg dosages. The tablets are usually scored down the middle so you can break them in half easily. You can break the halves in half too, to get the exact amount you want. An inexpensive pill-cutter may be useful for this purpose.

Remember, if a niacin tablet is taken on an empty stomach, a flush will occur (if it is going to occur at all) within about thirty minutes, usually sooner. If niacin is taken right after a meal, a flush may be delayed. In fact, the flush may occur long enough afterward that you forgot that you took the niacin! Don't let the flush surprise you. Remember that niacin does this, and you can monitor it easily.

You can powder the niacin tablet if you want a flush right away. This is easily done by crushing it between two spoons. Powdered niacin on an empty stomach can result in a flush within minutes. Take it with a hot beverage and the flush will occur even sooner. Niacin is heat-stable, so the temperature of food will not affect it at all.

Dr. Hoffer reported that side effects that may occur with really high doses of niacin are partly or largely offset by taking large doses of vitamin C. Hoffer had his patients take at least as much C as niacin. More vitamin C works even better. We have already mentioned the most common side effects: the flush, of course, and possibly nausea if you take way too much. Side effects tend to be more common in people with a history of liver disease and/or substantial alcohol use, commonly believed to be indicated by elevation of liver function tests. We will discuss this and other niacin side effects in the next chapter.

It is a good idea to take all the other B-complex vitamins in a separate supplement in addition to the niacin. The B vitamins, like professional baseball players, work best as a team. Still, the body seems to need proportionally more niacin than the other B vitamins. Even the U.S. Recommended Dietary Allowance (RDA) for niacin is much more than for any other B vitamin. Orthomolecular (nutritional) physicians consider the current RDA for niacin of only 18 mg or less to be way too low for optimum health. While the powers that be continue to discuss this, it is possible to decide for yourself based on the success of doctors who use niacin for their patients every day.

CHAPTER 5

Safety of Niacin

A doctor must know niacin in order to use it.
—WILLIAM PARSONS JR., M.D.

Pharmakon is an ancient Greek word that means both a remedy and a poison. It aptly describes drugs, but not orthomolecular substances like vitamins. Vitamins have established an excellent safety record, and this allows a very large margin for error. Still, there is a right way and a wrong way to do anything. In this chapter we will address the safety of vitamin B$_3$ therapy.

DOES NIACIN RAISE BLOOD SUGAR?

Sometimes it does. Many decades ago I (AH) began giving niacin to all my diabetic patients to keep their cholesterol levels normal and to decrease the serious vascular side effects of diabetes that lead to blindness and loss of legs. I did not see that many, but none of my diabetic patients on niacin suffered from those side effects. Their eyes remained normal as did their circulatory system. Many physicians had the idea that because niacin increased blood glucose levels in some patients that this was contraindication. However, that increase was usually minor and the patients did not suffer from those slight elevations. I found that one-third of my diabetic patients had to increase insulin levels a little, one-third had to *decrease* it, and the rest did not need to make any change.

Studies on Niacin and Blood Sugar

In a 1987 study by Vague et al., juvenile diabetics were given three grams (3,000 milligrams [mg]) of niacin per day. That dosage produced remissions in a large proportion of these young patients. The report on this study concluded, "Our results and those from animal experiments indicate that, in Type I diabetes, nicotinamide slows down the destruction of B cells and enhances their regeneration, thus extending remission time."[1]

In 2006, Canner et al. reported that niacin was valuable in treating post-infarction patients, whether or not they had the sugar metabolic syndrome. They did not find that niacin was contraindicated.[2] Similarly, Dube et al. reported that extended-release niacin "in doses up to 2,000 mg daily was safe, well-tolerated, and efficacious in HIV-infected subjects with athero-genic dyslipidaemia. Increases in glycaemia and insulin resistance tended to be transient."[3]

Kirkey reported the results of a study, published in *The Lancet* in 2008, that concluded that most people with diabetes should be taking statins. Kirkey's headline is a bit more intelligent, for she writes, "Diabetics should take cholesterol-lowering drugs,"[4] which of course would include niacin. You can visualize how much more therapeutic niacin will be if the statins, which are only a very poor distant cousin in effectiveness to niacin, were helpful. The statins only lower total cholesterol, do not elevate HDL, do not lower triglycerides, and do not lower lipoprotein(a). The statins decrease the least important metabolic factor, which has little relationship to heart disease and which does not extend life as niacin does. Abnormal-ity in blood lipid levels are main components of this cardiovascular syn-drome, which is also associated with decreased sugar tolerance and obesity. Since the main pathological side effects are changes in blood lipids and arteriosclerosis, niacin, which normalizes blood cholesterol levels, should theoretically be an important constituent of any treatment program for this condition and for type 1 and type 2 diabetes. Giving people niacin must be a most important treatment if we are to decrease the major pathol-ogy that both of these serious diseases generate.

But not everyone knows this. Here is an example of just how far irra-tionality seeps into medicine. In one study by Zhou et al.,[5] the authors claim that a mere 100 mg of niacinamide raises blood sugar. This is contrary to common sense, as well as contrary to Dr. Hoffer's extensive clinical experi-ence. He found that several thousand mg daily, long-term, raised blood sugar only slightly if at all. Another study by Li et al.[6] borders on the comical. After looking at blood glucose levels in exactly five people, the authors con-clude that niacin . . . contained in fortified foods! . . . is a cause of childhood obesity. How so? The authors claim that niacin stimulates appetite. How much niacin? This is the funniest part: they are talking single-digit RDA-levels—far, far less than even 100 mg. Might it be more likely that, just possibly, the cause of childhood obesity is overconsumption of fat and sugar? Perhaps the McNothing meals kids eat, or their huge consumption of soda, or lack of exercise? We think that observations on the blood glucose levels of five people are hardly the basis for reconsideration of niacin levels for a whole country. Research like this does not pass the straight-faced test.

Does Niacin Cause Macular Edema?

Rarely. Niacin can sometimes cause cystoid macular edema (spaces of fluid that form within the retina). This condition is unusual and completely reversible. Such changes are obvious in a standard retinal fundus exam when the patient reports symptoms of a visual deficit.[7]

This maculopathy is not associated with the characteristic leakage from retinal arterioles caused by diabetic retinopathy, as it goes away when niacin is discontinued or the dosage is reduced. There is a threshold dose.[8] Some case reports show that going from 3,000 mg/day down to 1,000–1,500 mg reverses the cystoid maculopathy.[7] The critical dose is likely to be related to the body weight, so that smaller people would have a lower threshold and larger people a higher figure. The reversibility and ease of detection factors are very important to niacin users. Persons taking niacin should note any changes in their vision, especially in reading, which uses the fovea and macula. Of those people taking niacin at high doses, only those that report visual symptoms need to be evaluated by an ophthalmologist.[9] The rate is very low, less than 1% of those taking high doses of niacin for reducing cholesterol.[7]

Some papers on this topic[10,11] offer authors' assessments of ocular side effects from herbals and nutritional supplements which seem a little alarmist, potentially leading the reader to generalize from the specific problems described in the article to an overall conclusion that nutrients and herbal supplements will inevitably lead to problems with toxicity. That is not the case. It is important that people understand that the side effects of niacin are specific to the patient's prior conditions and to the dose. People will notice if they develop eye problems. Because the side effects of niacin are reversible and easy to detect, this is a small and manageable problem. If those people taking supplements know that niacin has been reported in rare cases to cause eye problems, and that the problems are reversible, this will point them and their medical professionals in the right direction.

DOES NIACIN CAUSE LOW BLOOD PRESSURE?

Somewhat, but with qualifications. Generally speaking, supplemental niacin does not lower blood pressure very much if at all, and it is probably not a first-line therapy for essential hypertension. Dr. Hoffer's standard niacin prescription for his psychiatric patients was 3,000 mg per day in divided doses. People requiring more were gradually acclimated to an increase. He reported no hypotension in the thousands and thousands of patients he treated during more than half a century of medical practice.

Studies on the Relationship between Niacin and Blood Pressure

It is possible that a sudden, excessively large (over 5,000 mg at one time) dose may sometimes cause an abrupt drop in blood pressure. This is another good reason why self-administration of irrationally huge amounts of niacin is inappropriate. We again state that persons should obtain their physician's participation when using high doses.[12]

It is precisely because of this dramatic acute effect that niacin has been considered as a long-term blood-pressure-lowering agent. A 2009 placebo-controlled study of 1,613 men and women showed that extended-release niacin was associated with significant reductions in systolic blood pressure (SBP) and diastolic blood pressure (DBP) after twenty-four weeks. Reductions were not large: only about two to three mm Hg for either SBP or DBP.[13]

Another paper said that "Small clinical trials of acute niacin administration have shown significant BP-lowering effects of niacin in patients with hypertension but not necessarily in normotensive individuals. . . . Most large, prospective, randomised clinical trials involving niacin and niacin-containing regimens showed either no clear significant effects of niacin or slightly lower mean BP among some niacin treatment groups compared with placebo." The authors also wrote that "Larger studies, such as the Coronary Drug Project, suggest that niacin may lower BP when administered over a longer period of time."[14]

Common-sense caution applies: use niacin in cooperation with your doctor. In order to get such cooperation, be sure your doctor reads this next section first.

TOXICOLOGY

Vitamins are not toxic. Xenobiotics (drugs) are toxic. There is therefore no toxicology for vitamins. When taken in enormous amounts like water they can have undesirable side effects, but there are virtually no deaths associated with vitamins. I (AH) use this term because in spite of all the evidence that vitamins are safe and nontoxic, and in spite of the fact there is no evidence that they are toxic, most physicians still believe that niacin especially is toxic—simply because of its vasodilatory effect, the flush that occurs when it is first taken. This has been a bonanza for the drug companies, who are spending barrels of money trying to find a compound that they can patent that works as well as niacin for cholesterol management. They are looking for substances that will moderate the niacin flush. This is bizarre, since the best anti-flush product is niacin itself. *With continued use, very few patients still flush.* I have been taking 3,000 mg and more niacin daily for over fifty years and will, on occasion, have a mild flush (which I can feel but no one can see) if I have missed one dose.

Niacin Does Not Cause Liver Damage

One reader wrote: "I am megadosing on niacin and my liver function tests are elevated. So now, my doctor has told me to stop taking niacin. Just how significant are these liver function changes, anyway?"

The myth that niacin causes liver damage was thoroughly debunked by Dr. William B. Parsons Jr. in his book on niacin and cholesterol, *Cholesterol Control Without Diet! The Niacin Solution.*[15] The book discusses this problem extremely well. (A review can be found in *Journal of Orthomolecular Medicine,* Volume 14, 1999, 3rd quarter.) We consider Dr. Parsons to have been the most knowledgeable physician when it comes to treating patients with lipid problems using drugs and niacin. It is clear that he favors the use of niacin, not the drugs. He was the first physician outside of Saskatchewan, Canada to use niacin. He instigated the first niacin cholesterol studies and with his associates corroborated the claims that niacin lowered cholesterol made by Dr. Alshul, Dr. Stephen, and me (AH) in 1955. This discovery might have languished and never been rediscovered had we not gotten this corroboration from the prestigious Mayo Clinic, where Dr. Parsons was chief resident.

Dr. Parsons provides the evidence, based upon his own studies and the vast literature available, that using niacin to lower elevated cholesterol levels is the only practical, effective, safe, and cost effective method for

No Deaths from Niacin (or Any Other Vitamin): Poison Control Statistics Prove Supplements' Safety[16]

There was not even one death caused by a dietary supplement in 2009, according to the most recent information collected by the U.S. National Poison Data System.

The 200-page annual report of the American Association of Poison Control Centers, published in the journal *Clinical Toxicology,* shows zero deaths from multiple vitamins; zero deaths from any of the B vitamins; zero deaths from vitamins A, C, D, or E; and zero deaths from any other vitamin.

Additionally, there were no deaths whatsoever from any amino acid, herb, or dietary mineral supplement.

Two people died from non-nutritional mineral poisoning, one from a sodium salt and one from an iron salt or iron. On page 1139, the AAPCC report specifically indicates that the iron fatality was not from a nutritional supplement. One other person is alleged to have died from an "unknown dietary supplement or homeopathic agent." This claim remains speculative, as no verification information was provided.

Sixty poison centers provide coast-to-coast data for the U.S. National Poison Data System, "one of the few real-time national surveillance systems in existence, providing a model public health surveillance system for all types of exposures, public health event identification, resilience response and situational awareness tracking."

Over half of the population in the United States takes daily nutritional supplements. Even if each of those people took only one single tablet daily, that makes 155,000,000 individual doses per day, for a total of nearly 57 billion doses annually. Since many persons take more than just one vitamin or mineral tablet, actual consumption is considerably higher, and the safety of nutritional supplements is all the more remarkable.

If nutritional supplements are allegedly so "dangerous," as the U.S. Food and Drug Administration and news media so often claim, then *where are the bodies?*

The full text article is available for free download at http://www.aapcc.org/dnn/Portals/0/2009%20AR.pdf

Download any Annual Report of the American Association of Poison Control Centers from 1983–2009 free of charge at http://www.aapcc.org/dnn/NPDSPoisonData/NPDSAnnualReports.aspx

restoring lipid levels to normal. Niacin does more than decrease levels of low-density cholesterol. It elevates HDL, decreases lipoprotein(a) [Lp(a)], and lowers triglycerides. In comparison with the statins, it is the clear winner. And, it decreases mortality and extends life even after patients have already suffered their first coronary.

Niacin is a vitamin, not a drug. In addition to its effect on the lipid blood profile, it has the usual positive vitamin properties of megadose vitamin B3. Most physicians do not really know niacin since it is not patented, has no solicitous parent corporation to promote it, and is not advertised. It is difficult to pick up a medical journal without seeing some statin ads. I still have not seen one ad extolling the virtues of niacin. Since many physicians do not know niacin, they are suspicious of it. I find exasperating the total ignorance of niacin and the fear it generates. The medical profession is afraid that niacin is liver hepatotoxic, which it is not. Dr. Parsons points out that increases in liver function tests, unless they are very substantial, such as more than threefold, usually does not indicate liver pathology. There are many compounds that elevate liver enzymes—all the statins do, as do acetaminophen (Tylenol) and ibuprofen (Advil).

A second acceptance problem is the flush that accompanies niacin when one first starts to use it. Physicians who understand this and know how to work with it seldom have a problem, and their patients get along well with it. However, physicians who do not know anything about it tend to impart their lack of knowledge to their patients, who soon stop using it. According to Parsons, inositol hexaniacinate, the usual no-flush niacin in health food stores, is not nearly as good for lowering cholesterol, although it is as good for other conditions in which niacin is helpful, including psychoses, schizophrenia, and anxiety.

Since I (AH) began using megadoses of vitamin B3 in 1952, I have seen a few cases of obstructive-type jaundice that cleared up when the niacin was stopped. In one case I had to resume the use of niacin because the patient's schizophrenia recurred. He recovered and the jaundice did not recur. I have seen so few cases of jaundice that there is little evidence that the jaundice arose from the use of the niacin. Jaundice has a natural occurrence rate, and within any series of patients, a few will get jaundice from other factors. In rare cases, too much niacin causes nausea and vomiting, and if this persists because the niacin is not decreased or stopped then dehydration might become a factor. I have seen no cases of this in the past fifteen years. The main danger from taking niacin is not jaundice—it is that people will live longer.

Again we say: niacin is not liver toxic. That is a myth. This myth, which is pervasive in medicine, is based upon a series of observations, some of which were dead wrong. Between 1940 and 1950, when the toxicity of niacin and niacinamide were studied, the LD_{50} (lethal dose, 50%) of rats was determined. The LD_{50} is the amount of compound that will kill one half of the population of animals used to test toxicity. If 100 mice are given the drug and half die, that dose is the LD_{50}. For niacin the LD_{50} is very high, about 4.5 grams per kilogram. This is equivalent to 225 grams (nearly half a pound) for a 110 pound female and 360 grams for a 176 pound male, approximately 100 times the normal recommendation. Whether anyone will ever find an LD_{50} for people is extremely unlikely. At necropsy, the animals in the early studies of B_3 toxicity showed elevated fatty acids in the liver.

In 1950, deficiency of methyl groups was a popular topic. It was accepted that this deficiency caused fatty livers. Niacin and niacinamide are methyl acceptors, so it made sense to consider that too much vitamin B_3 would cause fatty acid livers by producing a methyl deficiency syndrome. However, Professor R. Altschul at the University of Saskatchewan could not confirm these findings. In his animal studies he found that the vitamin had no effect on the fatty-acid levels in the liver.

The second observation, which is still routinely made, is that niacin will increase liver function tests in some patients. It is assumed, incorrectly, that elevated liver function tests always mean underlying liver pathology. Many other medicines cause the same elevations of liver function tests. Usually after a few days off niacin the test results become normal. Therefore it is best to stop the niacin for five days and then do the tests to avoid confusing liver damage with increased liver function activity.

The Mayo Clinic used the electron microscope to examine the livers of a series of their patients on niacin being treated for high blood cholesterol. They found no evidence of pathology. This was first reported by Dr. William Parsons Jr. As mentioned above, Parsons points out that increases in the liver function tests do not indicate liver pathology unless they are very substantial. There are many compounds that elevate liver enzymes including all the statins. In most patients with elevated liver function tests, the values become normal in a few days even if the niacin is not discontinued.

I advise doctors that they should stop the niacin for at least five days before doing a liver function test. With real liver pathology, the results will not become normal in five days, but when they are elevated due to niacin, they will be normal within these five days. Liver enzymes are commonly elevated by many modern drugs. Gonzalez-Heydrich et al.[17] gave twelve children a combination of olanzapine and divalproic acid. Every one had an elevated enzyme peak, and in five it remained elevated for many months. Two children had to be removed from the study because of severe pathology, pancreatitis in one child and steatohepatitis in the other.

Over forty years ago there were a few reports of liver damage and one or two deaths caused by niacin and/or niacinamide. These were traced to poorly made slow-release preparations, not to standard preparations. I've used niacin for lowering cholesterol and both forms for treating schizophrenic patients since 1953, and have treated thousands of patients. Very few patients became jaundiced. As mentioned above, one patient recovering from schizophrenia on niacin became jaundiced. When the niacin was stopped, the jaundice cleared, but his schizophrenia came back. When the niacin was resumed, his schizophrenia cleared again, and the jaundice did not recur. I have seen no cases of jaundice in the past twenty years. But it is possible that the liver function test results may be raised due to methyl depletion. According to Dr. David Capuzzi, a specialist in diabetes, metabolism, and endocrinology in Philadelphia and one of the world's authorities on niacin and cholesterol, this can be prevented by giving patients 2,400 milligrams of lecithin divided twice daily. Betaine may also be effective for this purpose.

It is uncommon, but another possible side effect of high-dose niacin use is increased gastric acidity. This is probably because niacin stimulates the secretion of gastric juice.

Does Niacin "Mask" Tests for Illegal Drugs?

The answer is no. In a personal communication with niacin researcher Todd Pemberthy on this topic, he says, "'Masking' claims would appear to describe attempts to interfere with drug test assays. Niacin does not do this. The belief that any pill somehow masks a drug test indicates a lack of understanding of such tests."

However, Dr. Penberthy adds, "Niacin is without a doubt a powerful detoxifying agent. For example, when we are exposed to toxic environmental chemicals or cigarette smoke, there is a tremendous increase the expression of certain P450 enzymes, particularly CYP1A1. This is especially true in response to PCBs. PCBs and some other inducers are known to cause so much CYP1A1 to be made that it can comprise 10 percent of a liver cell's total protein, and that is a lot. Ultimately, this leads to a situation where you have boatloads of substrate and enzyme, but not necessarily a needed cofactor. The rate of any enzyme-catalyzed reaction is proportional to the concentrations of everything involved in the reaction, i.e. the substrate, enzyme, and cofactor. One key cofactor is derived from niacin: NADPH (Nicotinamide adenine dinucleotide phosphate). It is very important and used for many reactions; indeed, hundreds of proteins use NADPH. We need more niacin to make more NADPH."

A new review indicates that there have been quite a few niacin detoxification studies. (Niacin for detoxification: A little-known therapeutic use. *J Orthomolecular Med* 2011, 26: 2, 85–92). Detoxification is further discussed in Chapter 11 of this book.

Darkening of Skin

In rare instances, high-dose niacin can cause increased brown pigmentation of certain areas of the skin, usually the flexor surfaces (the skin in the underside of a joint). This is *not* acanthosis nigricans, even though it has been erroneously labeled as such. This is never a problem for patients if they are told the truth about what is occurring, but it is a problem for some doctors who are not familiar with it. This niacin-related reaction is a harmless pigmentation change, unlike acanthosis nigricans, which is a very serious, almost cancer-like condition. Dr. William Parsons Jr. correctly called it a skin change which *resembles* acanthosis nigricans. It does, but only in color, not in pathology. The browning effect of niacin in a very few subjects is entirely different. It is transient, usually lasting only a few months, and when it is clear the skin is perfectly normal. Like an old tan, it washes off if the skin is rubbed when moist. It never recurs even with continued use of niacin. I think it is due to the deposition of melanin-containing indoles from tyrosine and adrenalin. It occurs most commonly in schizophrenic patients and is part of the healing process.

It May Be Some Kind of Record, But Don't Do It

A young female teen-aged schizophrenic patient was given a month's supply of niacin, 200 tablets, each 500 mg. She became angry at her mother and the next day swallowed the whole bottle. For three days afterward, she had a sore abdomen but no other side effects. Another teen schizophrenic, after reading a paperback book on megavitamins and schizophrenia, could not find any physician to monitor her. She began to increase the dose on her own, and when she reached 60 grams (60,000 mg) niacin daily, all the voices she was hearing stopped. Two years later her maintenance dose was 3 grams (3,000 mg) per day. However, these are very extreme situations. Most people would have flushed severely, or would have been very nauseous, long before they got near such exorbitant doses. The take-home lesson is this: Even though niacin is safer than almost all over-the-counter drugs, you need to use good judgment. First, be informed. Second, work out your personal dose in cooperation with your doctor. And, whenever you notice a reaction that is unpleasant or worrying, contact your physician.

What About Negative News Media Comments About Vitamins?

Nutritional information that does make news generally stays far from the headlines, unless, of course, it is critical of vitamins. The most widely publicized vitamin therapy trials tend to be low-dose, worthless, negative, or all three. Mass media attention to a given nutritional research study appears to be inversely proportional to its curative value. Therefore, the public and not a few physicians remain unaware of the power of simple and safe natural methods, due to contradictory, inadequate, or just plain biased media reporting. When the press touts the "dangers" of vitamin "megadoses" while simultaneously overlooking Ritalin's carcinogenic potential, it strains at a gnat and swallows a camel. While drug side effects fill the *Physician's Desk Reference* to bursting, I think we could truly say that the chief side effect of vitamins is failure to take enough of them. Perhaps the very concept of "megadose" needs to be rethought, and re-presented to the public. The quantity of a nutritional supplement that cures an illness indicates the patient's degree of deficiency. It is therefore not a megadose of the vitamin but rather a megad-

No Deaths from Vitamins—None at All in 27 Years[18]

Over a twenty-seven year period, vitamin supplements have been alleged to have caused the deaths of a total of eleven people in the United States. A new analysis of US poison control center annual report data indicates that there have, in fact, been no deaths whatsoever from vitamins . . . none at all, in the twenty-seven years that such reports have been available.

The American Association of Poison Control Centers (AAPCC) attributes annual deaths to vitamins as:

2009: zero	2002: one	1995: zero	1988: zero
2008: zero	2001: zero	1994: zero	1987: one
2007: zero	2000: zero	1993: one	1986: zero
2006: one	1999: zero	1992: zero	1985: zero
2005: zero	1998: zero	1991: two	1984: zero
2004: two	1997: zero	1990: one	1983: zero
2003: two	1996: zero	1989: zero	

Even if these figures are taken as correct, and even if they include intentional and accidental misuse, the number of alleged vitamin fatalities is strikingly low, averaging less than one death per year for over two and a half decades. In 19 of those 27 years, AAPCC reports that there was not one single death due to vitamins. [1]

Still, one cannot help but be curious: Did eleven people really die from vitamins? And if so, how?

Vitamins Not *THE* Cause of Death

In determining cause of death, AAPCC uses a four-point scale called Relative Contribution to Fatality (RCF). A rating of 1 means "Undoubtedly Responsible"; 2 means "Probably Responsible"; 3 means "Contributory"; and 4 means "Probably Not Responsible." In examining poison control data for the year 2006, listing one vitamin death, it was seen that the vitamin's Relative Contribution to Fatality (RCF) was a 4. Since a score of "4" means "Probably Not Responsible," it quite negates the claim that a person died from a vitamin in 2006.

Vitamins Not *A* Cause of Death

In the other seven years reporting one or more of the remaining ten alleged vitamin fatalities, studying the AAPCC reports reveals an absence of any RCF rating for vitamins in any of those years. If there is no Relative Contribution to Fatality at all, then the substance did not contribute to death at all.

Furthermore, in each of those remaining seven years, there is no substantiation provided to demonstrate that any vitamin was a cause of death.

If there is insufficient information about the cause of death to make a clear-cut declaration of cause, then subsequent assertions that vitamins cause deaths are not evidence-based. Although vitamin supplements have often been blamed for causing fatalities, there is no evidence to back up this allegation.

The full text article is available for free download at http://www.aapcc.org/dnn/Portals/0/2009%20AR.pdf

Download any Annual Report of the American Association of Poison Control Centers from 1983–2009 free of charge at http://www.aapcc.org/dnn/NPDSPoisonData/NPDSAnnualReports.aspx The "Vitamin" category is usually near the very end of the report.

Special thanks to Jagan N. Vaman, M.D. for researching this article, which first appeared via the Orthomolecular Medicine News Service, June 14, 2011. All OMNS releases are archived for free access at http://www.orthomolecular.org/resources/omns/index.shtml.

eficiency of the nutrient that we are dealing with. A dry sponge holds more milk.

About half of the population of the United States and Canada takes vitamin supplements, even though the press often publishes some rather lurid accounts of how "dangerous" they can be. Note they do not write "will be," because there are no dead bodies strewn all over the landscape, as one might expect from such irresponsible news releases. Negative vitamin reporting is too often based on shoddy and almost fraudulent reports in medical journals, which are heavily subsidized by the pharmaceutical industry. It has been said that 80 percent of the studies in medical journals are wrong. Is this an underestimate?

What About Negative Medical Journal Vitamin Studies?

No mere estimates are involved here—there is clear evidence that the major medical journals are heavily influenced by their advertisers. A 2008 study showed that journals with the most pharmaceutical ads have the most negative reports about vitamins. The authors wrote that "In major medical journals, more pharmaceutical advertising is associated with publishing fewer articles about dietary supplements" and that journals with more pharmaceutical advertising had more articles with "negative conclusions about dietary supplement safety."[19] The following journals were specifically named as having the most pharmaceutical ads and the most negative articles about vitamins: the *Journal of the American Medical Association, New England Journal of Medicine, British Medical Journal, Canadian Medical Association Journal, Annals of Internal Medicine, Archives of Internal Medicine, Archives of Pediatric and Adolescent Medicine, Pediatrics and Pediatric Research,* and *American Family Physician.*

The results were statistically significant. Medical "journals with the most pharmads published no clinical trials or cohort studies about supplements. The percentage of major articles concluding that supplements were unsafe was 4 percent in journals with fewest and 67 percent among those with the most pharmads." The authors said that "the impact of advertising on publications" is real, and that "the ultimate impact of this bias on professional guidelines, health care, and health policy is a matter of great public concern."[20]

The flip side of this problem is that medical research and the very data it generates is biased by pharmaceutical advertising cash. The *Washington Post* reported that "Drug studies skewed toward study sponsors. Industry-funded research often favors patent-holders, study finds."[21]

In the *American Journal of Psychiatry* study the *Post* was referring to, the authors said, "In 90.0% of the studies, the reported overall outcome was in favor of the sponsor's drug. . . . On the basis of these contrasting findings in head-to-head trials, it appears that whichever company sponsors the trial produces the better antipsychotic drug."[22]

Even the former editor-in-chief of the *New England Journal of Medicine* agrees. Dr. Marcia Angell says, "Is there some way [drug] companies can rig clinical trials to make their drugs look better than they are? Unfortunately, the answer is yes. Trials can be rigged in a dozen ways, and it happens all the time. . . . [One of the] common ways to bias trials is to present only part of the data—the part that makes the product look good—and ignore the rest." She adds, "Bias is now rampant in drug trials. . . [Pharmaceutical] industry-sponsored research was nearly four times as likely to be favorable to the company's product as NIH [National Institutes of Health]-sponsored research. . . . The most dramatic form of bias is out-and-out suppression of negative results."[23]

This bias extends deeply into the medical schools themselves. Too many of tomorrow's doctors are bought and paid for with drug company money.

Dr. Angell writes, "Columbia University, which patented the technology used in the manufacture of Epogen and Cerezyme, collected nearly $300 million in royalties" in 17 years. "The patent was based on NIH-funded research." The U.S. National Institutes of Health gets its money from . . . you guessed it: your taxes. And, Dr. Angell adds, "In Harvard Medical School's Dean's Report for 2003–4, the list of benefactors included about a dozen of the largest drug companies. . . . The combined profits for the ten drug companies in the Fortune 500 were more than the profits for all the other 490 businesses put together."[24]

The *Washington Post* article quoted above said: "When the federal government recently compared a broader range of drugs in typical schizophrenia patients in a lengthy trial, the two medications that stood out were cheaper drugs not under patent."[25] Niacin works even better, and is cheaper, too. Niacin is a clinically proven therapy for serious mental illness, and yet the medical profession has refused to recommend it for over half a century.

Yet drugs are not the answer. A double-blind study of schizophrenics showed that three-quarters of them stopped taking their pharmaceutical medication, either because the drug's side effects were unbearable, or the drug just plain did not work.[26]

The Orthomolecular Medicine News Service commented, "Perhaps drugs are not the answer because mental illness is not caused by drug deficiency. But much illness, especially mental illness, may indeed be caused by nutrient deficiency or nutrient dependency. Only nutrients can correct this problem. This not only makes sense, it has stood up to clinical trial again and again. Vitamins like niacin are cheap, safe and effective. Modern "wonder drugs" are none of those. But they do make money. Especially when the drug makers control the research, the advertising, and the doctors. No wonder which approach you've heard more about."[27]

Most Niacin Side Effects Are Positive

If a patient takes niacin to normalize mental function, and as a result of the vitamin activity feels very much better in other areas such as more energy and faster healing, then this is a positive side effect. There are other positive side effects that often occur. For example, if the patient takes niacin to deal with his arthritis and at the same time his cholesterol levels decease, this result would be a major positive side effect or, better still, side benefit. Niacin lowers C-reactive protein (CRP), one of the markers of inflammation. The statins also lower CRP but, in contrast to the statins, niacin is not toxic.

Is Niacin Too Good to Be True?

There is a recurrent problem with vitamins being perceived as "too useful." Frederick R. Klenner, M.D., found vitamin C to be an effective and nearly all-purpose antitoxin, antibiotic, and antiviral. One vitamin curing polio, pneumonia, measles, strep, snakebite, and Rocky Mountain spotted fever? Laypeople and professionals alike certainly struggle with that, and more so with the fact that Klenner also reported success with nearly four dozen other diseases. How did he do it? The explanation may be as simple as this: the reason that one nutrient can cure so many different illnesses is because a deficiency of one nutrient can cause many different illnesses.

> Each year in the United States, well over 100,000 patients in hospitals die from drugs that are properly prescribed and taken as directed. The number of vitamin deaths per year is less than one. It is interesting how this fact stays out of the modern press.

This has led to something of a vitamin public relations problem. When pharmaceuticals are versatile, they are called "broad spectrum" and "wonder drugs." When vitamins are versatile, they are called "faddish" and "cures in search of a disease." Such a double standard needs to be exposed and opposed at every turn. Seemingly unrelated health problems may indeed be largely caused by a common nutritional deficiency. Treating accordingly was a good idea in the 1950s, when Dr. Hoffer was beginning his research. It is just as good today. Too good? We think this is a rather nice problem to have.

It is clear that vitamin B_3 is a very powerful yet benign substance that is involved in numerous reactions in the body, and which, in larger doses, is therapeutic and preventative for a large number of apparently unrelated diseases. It is highly likely that if any human community increases their population's intake of vitamin B_3 by even a few hundred milligrams per day (and to much higher levels in people already suffering from a number of pathological conditions), they will find a substantial decrease in mortality and an increase in longevity.

CHAPTER 6

Pandeficiency Disease

*Health is the fastest growing failing business
in western civilization.*
—EMANUEL CHERASKIN, M.D.

Doctors educated to dispense drugs using the "one drug, one disease" concept cannot understand any substance that is effective against more than one condition. It is looked upon as snake oil, not a real therapeutic compound, and one that is only a placebo. If our medical schools gave their medical students more than an hour or two of nutrition instruction for every four years of education (instead of so much surgery they will seldom do, or pathology they will leave to pathologists, or a whole lot of other material they will never use), students would graduate with a modern understanding that there is nothing more important than food and the proper intake of all the important nutrients to maintain and restore health and to fend off the invading organisms that look upon us as food. Of course they also seldom teach other important subjects such as the history of medicine, the patient-doctor relationship, and how to be a healers rather than merely laboratory-obsessed technicians taught to remember but not very often to think and reason. If they understood pellagra clinically— once a major scourge around the Mediterranean and the Southeastern United States—they would have a perfect example of how one simple compound, vitamin B_3, can cure a large number of conditions or disorders, diseases that apparently are not related to each other.

THE CONCEPT OF PANDEFICIENCY DISEASE

All the conditions we have found to be responsive to the orthomolecular program can be considered subsets of *pandeficiency disease,* a deficiency of several vitamins. The recent report by Marini[1] refers to a large number of mild to moderate enzyme problems that can be corrected by proper doses of the vitamins. The vitamins we use for all pandeficiency diseases are the B-complex vitamins, vitamin B_3 in much larger doses, vitamin C, selenium, often zinc, sometimes vitamin E, and omega-3 essential fatty acids. This suggests that these are the main vitamins and minerals that should be investigated and followed up. There may be no advantage in analyzing the personal genome at this moment in history, as these vitamins and minerals are relatively cheap and easily available. Marini wrote: "I wouldn't be surprised if everybody is going to require a different optimum dose of vitamins depending on their make up." No surprise was necessary. If he had been familiar with orthomolecular medicine, he would have anticipated this.

Pellagra is characterized by the four D's: dermatitis, diarrhea, dementia, and death. It is caused by a diet deficient in protein, essential fatty acids, and minerals and vitamins, especially B_3. It is cured by a good diet reinforced with the same vitamin.

Suppose a professor lectured to her medical students for one hour on skin lesions, one hour on gastrointestinal lesions, and one hour on psychoses . . . but did not tell her students that these were all symptoms of one disease called pellagra, which is caused by one deficiency. During her fourth lecture she tells the students that one vitamin cures all of these illnesses, without teaching them the concept of deficiency diseases and pellagra in particular. The students would be mystified, would probably think she was nuts, and certainly would have major difficulty understanding how one drug could be so versatile. This was the situation before serological tests became the diagnostic criterion for syphilis. It also expressed itself in many different ways. Old textbooks used forty or more pages of valuable space to describe its many symptoms and ways of treatment since there was no true treatment until penicillin came along. Now syphilis is rarely mentioned. It is diagnosed by a blood test and is treated by one drug. In times past, it was said that if you understood syphilis, you understood all of medicine. I think the same can be said about pellagra.

Diagnosis classifies disease for two main reasons: (1) to improve prognosis, and (2) to improve treatment. Prognosis is very important so patients and family can prepare for the future, especially if the future is very dim. Estimating when a person will die may be extremely important for all sorts of reasons. Before specific treatment was discovered, doctors were judged on their ability to prognose correctly. It would be very bad for the physician's reputation if his prognosis were wrong. Many years ago when I (AH) started to practice medicine, some of my patients, when giving me their history, would tell me that their doctor had told them they would die but the doctor died before they did. Good doctors were good prognosticators—and this depended upon accurate diagnosis.

Diagnosis became even more important when specific treatments were discovered. Diagnosis advised the clinician what treatment to use. It was assumed that patients with the same diagnosis would respond to a similar treatment already described by other doctors. I had pneumonia in my early teens. Our friendly family doctor (he was also surgeon, emergency doctor, obstetrician, and so on, as he was the only doctor in the community) told my mother I had pneumonia and ordered mustard plasters. It must have been very effective or else my pneumonia was very mild, as I was well in a couple of days. That was standard treatment for a disease that killed a large proportion of its victims. This type of diagnosis was a descriptive diagnosis. By listening to my chest the doctor discovered something wrong and concluded that it was most likely pneumonia. No other diagnostic tests were available.

After it was discovered that many different lung lesions were possible, it became necessary to distinguish one lesion from another. Was it bacterial, and if so, which bacteria, staph or strep? Today specific laboratory tests are used to determine this. Diagnosis is now etiologic—based on the cause of the condition. And until the causal diagnosis is made, the treatment cannot be very successful. This is the pathway diagnosis has traveled; from description of the site, the organ, and later to the cause when known. If the cause remains unknown, the diagnosis remains descriptive. Psychiatric diagnosis is almost entirely descriptive.

Medical schools teach medical students the use of medicines, not nutrients. From their nutrition lectures, if any, students will be told that only small amounts of niacin are ever needed by the human body, and that large doses do virtually nothing but result in "expensive urine." Yet it is widely known that a small amount of niacin prevents pellagra. It is less well-known that much larger doses of niacin cure the more dreadful symptoms of advanced pellagra: dermatitis, psychosis, dementia, diarrhea, and heart enlargement.

We willingly concede the successes of crisis medicine, while sticking to our guns that nutritional medicine is better for the prevention and treatment of chronic illness. Pharmaceutical medicine has a near-monopoly on healthcare service delivery. Such a monopoly probably results in more use of drugs than of nutrients.

Principles of Orthomolecular Nutrition

- Most nonaccidental illnesses are due to malnutrition. This not only includes chronic diseases, but also viral and bacterial acute illnesses, which are greatly aggravated by inadequate nutrition. Conventional physicians are valuable for persons needing treatment of traumatic injury.

- Adding pharmaceutical drugs to a sick body to cure it is like adding poison to a polluted lake to clean it. Killing microorganisms or masking the cause of symptoms is no more than a temporary answer in either case.

- Restoring health must be done nutritionally, not pharmacologically. All of our cells are made exclusively from what we drink and eat. Not one cell is made from a drug.

- Nutrient therapy increases individual resistance to disease. Drug therapy generally lowers resistance to disease. Healthy plants, healthy animals, and healthy people do not get sick. Doctors do not like to admit this, because healthy people do not go to doctors.

- The quantity of a nutritional supplement required to cure an illness indicates the patient's degree of deficiency. It is therefore not a megadose of the vitamin, but rather a megadeficiency of the nutrient that we are dealing with. Uncorrected deficiency leads to vitamin *dependency*.

- The number-one side effect of vitamins is failure to take enough of them.

- With vitamin therapy, speed of recovery is proportional to the dosage given. Just as there is a certain, large amount of fuel needed to launch an aircraft or a spacecraft, there is a certain, large amount of nutrients needed to cure a sick body.

- The reason one nutrient can cure so many different illnesses is because a deficiency of one nutrient can cause many different illnesses.

- In high doses, a nutrient can act as a drug, but a drug can never act as a nutrient.

- Vitamin supplementation is not the problem—it is undernutrition that is the problem. Vitamins are the solution.

- Nutritional therapy is inexpensive, effective, and, most important, safe. There is not even one death per year from vitamins. (See Chapter 4 for more about vitamin safety.)

The Role of Sugar, Diet, and, Uh, Constipation

During World War II, Royal Navy Surgeon Captain T. L. Cleave was concerned about the physical ill health of many of the sailors. From his studies he concluded that most of them suffered from one overall disease he called the "Saccharine Disease" in 1956[2]. The saccharine disease has no relation to the synthetic sweetener. Saccharine in this case refers to a detrimental craving for sweet tastes and consequent overuse of sugar. (And no, we do not recommend sugar substitutes. Artificial sugar substitutes have problems of their own, not the least of which is that they may stimulate people to want still more and more sweet foods.)

Cleave presented evidence that the various diseases of civilization are one disease, not a large number of discrete diseases.[3] I (AH) had a copy of his original publication, but it was worn out by constant use. This book turned my life around. I became a full-time nutritionist. Cleave's experience as a physician convinced him that overconsumption of sugar and processed carbohydrates was the root cause of diabetes, coronary disease, obesity, malabsorption, peptic ulcer, constipation, hemorrhoids, varicose veins, E. coli infections, appendicitis, cholicystitis, pyelitis, diverticulitis, renal calculus, many skin conditions, and dental caries.[4]

This nutritional disease affected all the organs and systems, which were then diagnosed and named according to the organ or malfunction of that organ. The cause is the modern diet, which is too rich in sugars and refined carbohydrates and too deficient in food containing its original fiber. It is also deficient in essential fatty acids, vitamins, and minerals, relating it to pandeficiency disease. This diet typically relies on refined cereals devoid of their bran and germ such as white bread, polished rice, and a heavy intake of sugar averaging about 125 pounds per person each year. Cleave did consider the role played by the deficiency of essential nutrient factors. He emphasized the excessive intake of sugar and the deficiency of fiber. In other words, he emphasized the value of whole foods.

The massive evidence Cleave presented had little impact, except for a sudden interest in bran as if it were a drug especially designed for people with constipation. Cleave did give his sailors bran, but he was much more concerned with the white flour they were eating. His message was clear: what was needed were the original whole grain cereals as in whole wheat and rice. Just adding bran only provided a partial answer. In 1972 Professor

John Yudkin published his book *Sweet and Dangerous*[5]. He presented the evidence that proved sugars were the culprit. His work was ignored.

Ever since reading Cleave's book many years ago, I have advised my patients to follow a sugar-free, refined carbohydrate-free diet. I think most of those who followed my advice have been grateful. There is nothing more pleasing than feeling good.

How could this one explanation account for such an amazing number of diseases? This is how: constipation is the main outcome of a diet deficient in fiber-rich foods, not in a simple deficiency of fiber. If it were a simple deficiency of fiber, one could eat fiber made from wood. This will certainly increase the fiber intake, but will do little for one's health. Chronic constipation leads to the other diseases of the intestine. In South Africa, it was said you had be English to get appendicitis—the natives, who still ate high fiber foods, did not. The remaining diseases come from high sugar intake. These are diabetes, coronary disease, and metabolic disease.

Everyone knows that the major problem with modern foods is that they are too high in fat. But is this really true? When I said "everyone," I was exaggerating; a few of us instead thought that too much sugar and not enough fiber-rich food were much more pathological. But the sugar industry was more adept at deflecting blame from their source of revenue, and the meat and fat industries were a bit lax in fighting and followed the same idea. Reviewing the recent evidence, Challem concluded that high-protein diets, still very controversial but more popular then they were when they were highlighted by Robert Atkins, helped people lose weight, improve their blood sugar levels, and normalize blood lipids.[6] Of three diets tested in Israel, the best results were obtained with the high-protein, high-fat diets. This included the levels of blood lipids. High cholesterol and high triglyceride levels do not come from high fat intake. They come from too much sugar. Again, stone-age diet advocates are vindicated.

The saccharine disease is also characterized by a deficiency in vitamins and minerals. The foods richest in these nutrients are not consumed. There is really no question about this, and it is well recognized by government as well as by the public. If governments concluded that diets were adequate they would not have mandated the addition of three vitamins and iron to white flour—and I would not have gotten my first job as a control chemist in a flour mill. Vitamin C, thiamine, riboflavin, niacinamide, vitamin D, iodine, and calcium are some of the nutrients that enrich our foods. But the most striking was the eradication of pellagra in the United States within two years after the addition of niacinamide to white flour was mandated in 1942. The Canadian government would not permit this. The American law was considered an adulteration by Canada, except that it had to ship the enriched flour overseas to the allied troops and the Canadian Commissioner of Indian Affairs insisted that it be given to Canadian natives who used it to make bannock (flat bread).

The enrichment of flour was one of the most beneficial public health measures ever, not only in preventing physical disease but in preventing mental disease. Before enriched flour became available, up to one-third of admissions to mental hospitals in the Southeastern United States were pellagrins, who could not be differentiated from schizophrenia by clinical examination alone. Pellagra—characterized by the four D's: dermatitis, diarrhea, dementia, and death—was gone. In the whole history of psychiatry, there has never been a public health measure as effective. The addition of a few pennies' worth of B_3 to flour saved the United States and the rest of the world billions of dollars of disease-generated costs. The addition of folic acid to flour has done the same.

Yes, the fortification of processed food was one of the most beneficial public health measures in history. Still, only *some* of the necessary nutrients are replaced by fortification. For this reason, we think it's important to reduce your carbohydrate intake, especially that of simple carbohydrates. The solution is a diet of unprocessed whole foods. Such a diet automatically provides much more fiber, more vitamins and minerals, and far less sugar. Nutritionists in the past and ever since have ignored the importance of this. It remains difficult for anyone to obtain an adequate intake of vitamins on a refined-carbohydrate dominated diet.

Roger Williams' demonstration that we are biochemically different has not been taken seriously by the medical and nutritional establishment even when they have been aware of it. This in spite of the fact we differ in our blood types, in our fingerprints, and more. The concept of individualization is so strong in our culture that nothing will stop people and make them stare more than three identical triplets walking down the street. I think that individualization is a key to the formation of the parent-infant relationship. And yet the worldwide nutritional standards do not take individuality into account. Indeed, standard-setters act as if we all have the same needs, except in a few clear-cut situations such as pregnancy. Recent research from the University of California at Berkeley provides a clear scientific explanation for what Williams hypothesized. Marini and colleagues reported in the *Proceedings of the National Academy of Sciences* that there are many genetic differences that make people's enzymes less efficient, and that simple supplementation with vitamins can restore some of these deficient enzymes to normal.[7] This work follows that of Bruce Ames, who found that you can cure genetic disease in babies by giving them vitamins.[8] Each person has a unique genome. It follows that all the clinical nutrition research over the past half a century where very small doses and a limited dose range were used have been a waste of money and time. They have also poisoned the attitude toward vitamins, except among the general population, over half of whom are taking them. Looks as if the scientists were wrong, but not the public. One day the genome may be used to determine which vitamins should be used, and how much. This work following Ames is itself a major follow-up of Linus Pauling and his concept of orthomolecular medicine. We in this field who have been practicing this concept, based upon clinical observations going back sixty years, are now bolstered by this research, which establishes the genetic mechanism for individuality.

In our book *Orthomolecular Nutrition*[9], we described some of the psychiatric symptoms associated with the saccharine disease, caused by excess sugar intake. These are anxiety and depression. The patients were referred to me by their family doctors because of these symptoms. When I first read about the role of hypoglycemia in causing mental disease, I was very skeptical, but I was also curious. A young female was referred to me for depression. She told me that her main problem was that she was frigid. Psychoanalysis was riding high many years ago, and it occurred to me that she would be a perfect candidate for psychoanalysis or deep psychotherapy to explore why she was having this problem. However, since I felt it was unlikely that this was caused by hypoglycemia, she would be ideal to disprove its effect. I ordered the five hour glucose tolerance test. The curve was typically hypoglycemic, to my surprise. She was equally surprised. Not expecting that it would help, I still advised her to avoid all sugar and increase her intake of protein. To my amazement, she was normal in one month. I was now more interested than skeptical. I began to routinely have patients with anxiety and depression take the test, and found that over 75 percent had the typical abnormal glucose tolerance curves. I no longer remained skeptical. Since then I have placed every patient on a sugar-free and refined-carbohydrate-free diet without doing any more tests. The condition was present in every one of three hundred alcoholics tested by the five hour glucose tolerance test. I did not realize it then, but sugar created disease by playing havoc with the metabolism of sugar, raising it up and down. Many patients are allergic to it. Other foods, like milk, to which patients are allergic will also give the typical glucose tolerance curves. Over the years I concluded that if every doctor who referred their patients to me were to test them and treat them with the special diet first, I would lose half of my psychiatric practice.

Indeed, whatever health problem you may have, sugar will make it worse. Health crusader Paul C. Bragg was right: "The best part of a donut is the hole." American's consumption of sucrose and high-fructose corn syrup grew from 127 pounds per person in 1986 to a teeth-chattering 153 pounds in 1996.[10] A sugar industry magazine advertisement from the 1970s that I (AWS) have says, "If sugar is fattening, why are kids so thin?" Perhaps the "fat" industries were too lax in competing with this message, and ultimately lost the information war. In the last two decades, people are, in fact, eating somewhat less fat and more sugar. And now, the envelope please: kids today are much fatter. Childhood obesity is epidemic. We can easily accept that the sugar industry was wrong. It is much more difficult to accept that the medical and nutrition professions backed the wrong horse.

The B Vitamins

Decades ago, Cleave considered the fact that the "saccharine disease" diet was also deficient in the B vitamins. Nutritionists since have ignored this, even though massive surveys have shown that it is impossible to obtain enough vitamin B with this diet. Nor did it occur to me (AH) until I had many more years of experience using large doses of the B vitamins. We treated schizophrenic patients with large doses of niacin or niacinamide and ascorbic acid. This treatment was based on our hypothesis that schizophrenia was caused by the excess conversion of adrenalin to adrenochrome, a product of oxidation. We used niacin to decrease the formation of adrenalin and ascorbic acid to inhibit its oxidation. Other catecholamines could also be oxidized in the body due to superoxidative stress. Over the following years it became clear that many other diseases also responded to increased doses of some of the vitamins. Eventually my objective in treating patients changed. I no longer aimed at just curing their disease; I was now interested in much more. I planned on giving them a multinutrient program that would not only help them get well but would keep them well until they died, as long as they remained on the program. Extra niacin remains one of the nutrients that is especially valuable.

Life extension also became an objective, as it had already been shown that niacin would decrease death and increase longevity. Finally, I concluded that I would no longer adhere to the one drug, one disease concept that permeates medicine and the drug industry. Instead, I would do what I could using nutrition and relevant nutrients to help patients regain their ability to deal with stress and with disease. People heal themselves if they are given the right tools with which to do so. I have been using the same therapeutic program for many years and have seen a large number of patients recover from different physical and mental disorders using it. In the same way that added sugar and refined carbohydrates will cause saccharine disease,[11] a multiple deficiency of vitamins will cause what I now call the pandeficiency disease. Pandeficiency disease is a general disorder that can affect any organ, system, or function, or any combination of them. About half of the population suffers from this chronic pervasive disease, caused by the overall deficiencies present in modern high-tech diets. If the psychiatric profession were to look carefully at the diagnostic system it now uses, it could eliminate hundreds of psychiatric disorders right along with their DSM numbers (*Diagnostic and Statistical Manual of Mental Disorders,* published by the American Psychiatric Association). Almost all of the ADD (attention deficit disorder) diagnoses of children could be eliminated.

In a recent editorial,[12] Dr. Sidney MacDonald Baker discusses the term "biomedical." He points out that with every patient there are two essential questions: (1) Does the person have a special need, and (2) Does he need to avoid or get rid of something to be healthy. It is a "get and get rid of" approach. Getting the question right is more valuable than trying to decide what the diagnosis is. Dr. Baker describes three main biochemical problems: detoxification, oxidative stress, and inflammation. These three factors describe the major diseases of modern civilization. He concludes "The term biomedical should convey a sense of rejection of the utter nonsense of at least one aspect of current mainstream medicine: the acceptance of the notion you can take a group of people who are sick in similar ways, give a descriptive name such as autism, colitis, depression, etc. to the group, and then say that the symptoms are caused by the name." The term pandeficiency should be considered a biomedical description.

The treatment of pandeficiency syndrome includes restoration of nutritious diet, attention to the intestinal flora, and the following few nutrients: vitamin B_3, both niacin and niacinamide, ascorbic acid, a strong B-complex preparation like 50 mg or 100 mg B-complex, selenium, zinc, calcium, magnesium, and omega-3 essential fatty acids. The doses depend on the symptomatology.

Access to Information, or Censorship?

These conclusions are based upon my (AH) personal experience in treating many patients with many conditions. I've described case histories, beginning in 1960, in 30 books and in 600 publications in the establishment press and in the alternative press, mostly in the *Journal of Orthomolecular Medicine* (*J Orthomolecular Med*). Curiously enough, forty-three years of *J Orthomolecular Med* have been blacked out by MEDLINE. Specifically, the taxpayer-supported U.S. National Library of Medicine refuses to index four decades of this peer-reviewed journal. Consequently, we consider MEDLINE to be the official censoring organization of the medical establishment. Our correspondence with NLM-MEDLINE confirmed that they actually do receive this journal by mail, but presumably keep it properly hidden in some dark closet and classified as top secret. But their censoring role is coming to an end, as Google and other search engines now provide easy access to *J Orthomolecular Med* papers.

In our (AH and Harold Foster) book, *Feel Better, Live Longer with Vitamin B_3*, we summarized the epidemiological literature and reviewed clinicians' experience in treating these vitamin-deficient conditions. Our conclusion was that about half of the population, the sick half, would benefit by taking extra vitamin B_3. About half of the population suffers from one or more chronic conditions. The fact that a nutrient, such as niacin, can act on more than one disease sometimes results in it not being taken seriously as therapy. It may be derided as "a cure in search of a disease" and dismissed out of hand.

Whether it is some kind of a conspiracy or not, it is clearly in the interests of pharmaceutical medicine to see that people continue to be advised that all the nutrition they need can be obtained from a regular, "balanced," unsupplemented diet. This official misinformation will likely continue until the public demands change.

The U.S. Recommended Dietary Allowance (RDA) for a given vitamin does not really apply to any specific person. Rather, it is a political judgment based on a theoretical average. And as RDAs demonstrate, the "average" is so low it resembles a mandated minimum wage that may never be exceeded. Should everyone work for minimum wage? Do we all really have pretty much the same nutritional needs? When is the last time you bought one-size-fits-all underwear that actually fit?

CHAPTER 7

Reversing Arthritis with Niacinamide: The Pioneering Work of William Kaufman, M.D., Ph.D.

*I noted that niacinamide (alone or combined
with other vitamins) in a thousand patient-years
of use has caused no adverse side effects.*
—WILLIAM KAUFMAN, M.D., PH.D.

Almost half the Canadian population older than seventy-five years has arthritis, and this illness is the third most common cause of disability in the country, costing some $4.8 billion each year. Dr. William Kaufman was the second orthomolecular physician inducted into the Orthomolecular Hall of Fame in 2004. He proved that large doses of niacinamide healed arthritis and many of the changes of aging. He used at least 2,000 milligrams (mg) per day, divided into four or even eight smaller doses daily. One would think that this important discovery would be taken very seriously. It was not, even though it has been confirmed by one controlled study and by physicians who has seen what has happened to their patients. This chapter summarizes the discoveries and writings of Dr. Kaufman regarding vitamin B$_3$ (niacinamide) and its beneficial effect on arthritis.

ARTHRITIS AND NIACINAMIDE

The world was still deep in the Great Depression when William Kaufman, M.D., Ph.D., had already begun treating osteoarthritis with two to four grams of niacinamide daily. Now, over seventy years later, his pioneering work in orthomolecular medicine is receiving the recognition it so well deserves.

In a 1978 radio interview with Carlton Fredericks, Dr. Kaufman described how "I had one patient who was so severely arthritic that I could not bend his elbows enough to measure his blood pressure. He was one of my first patients. I gave him niacinamide for a week in divided doses, and then he could bend his arm. I took him off it and gave him a look-alike medicine (placebo). In a week he was back where he was before: his joints were stiff again.

"I arrived at my (megavitamin B$_3$ dosage) schedule by actually seeing the response of patients with varying degrees of arthritis. One cannot give a single large dose and get any really favorable results in arthritis. . . . It is necessary to divide the doses, so that the blood levels of niacinamide would be fairly uniform throughout the waking day."

Kaufman's findings were both plain and elegant. The greater the stiffness, the more frequent the doses. Severely crippled arthritic patients needed up to a total of 4,000 mg per day, divided into ten doses per day. After one to three months of this treatment, patients could get out of their chair or bed. "If continued, they would be able to comb their hair and be able to walk upstairs, so they would no longer be prisoners of the house. By the end of about three years of treatment, they would be fully ambulatory, and this was even in the older age groups."

After being out of print for over sixty years, Dr. Kaufman's detailed clinical experience treating arthritis with megadoses of niacinamide has been posted in its entirety at http://www.doctoryourself.com and is freely available for online reading.

Special features of Dr. Kaufman's book include highly specific niacinamide dosage information applicable to both osteoarthritis and rheumatoid arthritis, along with the doctor's meticulous case notes for hundreds of patients, and some remarkably prescient observations on the antidepressant-antipsychotic properties of niacinamide. Kaufman, whom his widow has described as a conservative physician, nevertheless was the first to prescribe as much as 5,000 mg niacinamide daily, in many divided doses, to improve range of joint motion.

Dr. Kaufman's book, *The Common Form of Joint Dysfunction: Its Incidence and Treatment*, states:

> Theoretically, optimal nutrition must be continuously available to bodily tissues to ensure the best possible structure and function of tissues. While we do not know what constitutes optimal nutrition, it has been demonstrated empirically that even persons eating a good

or excellent diet according to present-day standards exhibit measurable impairment in ranges of joint movement which tends to be more severe with increasing age. It has also been demonstrated that when such persons supplement their good or excellent diets with adequate amounts of niacinamide, there is, in time, measurable improvement in ranges of joint movement, regardless of the patients' ages. In general, the extent of recovery from joint dysfunction of any given degree of severity depends largely on the duration of adequate niacinamide therapy.

Whenever a patient taking the amounts of niacinamide prescribed by the physician, and eating a good or excellent diet, fails to make satisfactory improvement in his Joint Range Index, in the absence of excessive mechanical joint injury the niacinamide schedule must be revised upward to that level which permits satisfactory improvement. Failure of the patient to take niacinamide as directed will result in failure to improve at a satisfactory rate.[1]

Chapter Overview of *The Common Form of Joint Dysfunction*

Dr. Kaufman's important book is worth reviewing in detail. We provide a brief summary of the contents below, and as mentioned above, the entire work is now available online. The book's 248 references are also posted at http://www.doctoryourself.com/kaufman11.html.

Chapter 1: Dr. Kaufman presents his niacinamide treatment protocol, beginning with his rationale and measurement methods. He also used ascorbic acid, thiamine, and riboflavin, all in large doses. There is a fascinating passage about "decreased running" (Attention Deficit Hyperactivity Disorder—ADHD). The chapter closes with case histories and an insightful, practical discussion of patient management.

Chapter 2: Dr. Kaufman discusses "Four Complicating Syndromes Frequently Coexisting with Joint Dysfunction," specifically physical and psychological stresses, allergy, posture, obesity, and other factors that may interact or interfere with niacinamide-megavitamin therapy for arthritis.

Chapter 3: "Coordination of Treatment" is a brief summary of Dr. Kaufman's practical recommendations for case management.

Chapter 4: The 42-page "Analysis of Clinical Data" contains Dr. Kaufman's meticulous patient records supporting megavitamin therapy with niacinamide. This statistical analysis contains fifty-three charts, tables, and graphs, which are not reproduced online.

Chapter 5: "Some Inferences Concerning Joint Dysfunction." Dr. Kaufman, writing in 1949, shows remarkable foresight of orthomolecular medicine half a century into the future. In this chapter he describes how the lack of a single nutrient can cause diverse diseases, the need for a new way of looking at arthritis, and reviews his treatment and what level of success to expect.

Hardcover copies of the original 1949 edition of Dr Kaufman's book (194 pages plus references) are available at www.doctoryourself.com.

Given Dr. Kaufman's work, the authors of a 1996 study on niacinamide and osteoarthritis, "The effect of niacinamide in osteoarthritis: a pilot study"[3] could have omitted the words "pilot study" from their title. Dr. William Kaufman had, forty-seven years earlier, already published his meticulous case notes for hundreds of patients, along with specific niacinamide dosage information applicable to both osteoarthritis and rheumatoid arthritis. In addition, the doctor added some remarkably prescient observations on the antidepressant-antipsychotic properties of B_3.

References to more of Dr. Kaufman's other writings can be found in the For Further Reading section at the end of this book.

In November 1999, Dan Lukaczer, N.D., reported in *Nutrition Science,* "A few years ago, Wayne Jonas et al. (1996) from the National Institutes of Health (NIH) Office of Alternative Medicine in Bethesda, MD, conducted a 12-week, double-blind, placebo-controlled study of 72 patients to assess the validity of Kaufman's earlier observations that niacin was of great benefit to the elderly, reducing arthritis. Jonas reported that niacinamide at 3 g/day reduced overall disease severity by 29 percent, inflammation by 22 percent and use of anti-inflammatory medication by 13 percent."[4] Patients in the placebo group either had no improvement or worsened.

Many of my (AH) patients with arthritis recovered or became much better when prescribed niacin.[5] The most dramatic case came into my office in a wheelchair, pushed by her very tired and sick-looking husband. She was sitting with her legs crossed over as she could not extend them. She had been sick for the previous twenty years and had received every known

Dr. William Kaufman's Notes on Niacinamide Therapy for Arthritis[1]

(Used with the kind permission of Charlotte Kaufman)

The (more frequent) 250 mg dose of niacinamide is 40 to 50 percent more effective in the treatment of arthritis than the (less frequent) 500 mg dose. As an illustration, see my Tom Spies Memorial Lecture: "Niacinamide, a Most Neglected Vitamin." This illustrative case history begins on page 17 column 2 and continues on page 18 column 2.

Do not use hard gelatin capsules containing 250 mg niacinamide because they do not deliver niacinamide as efficiently as 250mg niacinamide in thin gelatin capsules in the treatment of joint dysfunction (arthritis).

In my 1955 paper in the *Journal of the American Geriatrics Society*, I noted that niacinamide (alone or combined with other vitamins) in a thousand patient-years of use has caused no adverse side effects.[2]

Some brands of niacinamide on the market today contain excipients that act as preservatives, probably meant to prolong shelf life. Some patients have adverse reactions to these preparations, but most do not experience any ill effects.

Niacinamide has ungated entrance to the central nervous system. It has a strong affinity for the central nervous system's benzodiazepine receptors and causes a pleasant calmative effect. In addition, it improves central nervous system function in the kinds of central nervous symptom impairments noted in my 1943 book, starting on page 3.

Please keep in mind niacinamide is a systemic therapeutic agent. It measurably improves joint mobility, muscle strength, decreases fatigability. It increases maximal muscle working capacity, reduces or completely eliminates arthritic joint pain. Niacinamide heals broken strands of DNA and improves many kinds of CNS functioning.

Some joints are so injured by the arthritic process that no amount of niacinamide therapy will cause improvement in joint mobility, but it takes three months of niacinamide therapy before you can conclude this, since some joints are slow to heal.

treatment for arthritis, including hormones and gold injections. Nothing had helped. Her hands were totally useless and she was crippled. Her husband had to carry her around the house, even to the bathroom. He provided her with the equivalent care of four nurses, around the clock. No wonder he was totally exhausted and sick. I "knew" she could not be helped, since such very chronic deteriorated arthritis cases generally did not do well. She said to me, "I know that you cannot help my arthritis, but the pain in my back is terrible. All I want is some relief from it." I started her on a vitamin program, the main constituent of which was niacin, but I did not really expect to see much improvement. She returned a month later in her wheelchair, again being pushed by her husband. This time, however, she was sitting in her chair with her feet dangling straight down. Her husband looked relaxed and had lost his dreadful sick look. When I began to talk and ask her questions, she interrupted and said "The pain is gone!" She was so much better that I began to think that maybe, with skillful surgery, some function might be restored to her hands. Six months later she telephoned. I asked her in surprise, "How did you get to the phone?" She replied that she was now able to get around on her own in her chair, and added that she was not calling for herself but for her husband who had a cold. She wanted some advice about how to help him. This woman died several years later having achieved her goal of a pain-free existence.

From Hoffer and Foster:

> Arthritis recently has been at the centre of a vortex of controversy. In October 2004, Vioxx (rofecoxib), one of the main drugs used to treat it, was voluntarily withdrawn by its manufacturers, Merck and Co. It had been admitted that some 70,000 deaths, largely from cardiovascular episodes, had been associated with this drug's use. Such toxic side effects had been known by the industry for several years. In February 2005, a panel of the U.S. Food and Drug Administration voted to allow the possible return of Vioxx, provided it carried a striking black-box warning on its label about its cardiovascular risks. Patients who take it will be obliged to sign consent forms. 15 million prescriptions of Vioxx were filled in Canada before its withdrawal and it is not yet clear whether Health Canada will support its return to use. Interestingly, the *New York Times* reported that 10 of the 32 members of the U.S. Food and Drug Administration panel voting to allow the return of Vioxx were paid consultants for the drug's makers.[6] This panel also supported the continued use of other cox-2 drugs such as Celebrex and Bextra for arthritis despite their known cardiovascular risks, so long as they also carry a black-box warning. Given the evidence that arthritis can often be successfully treated with niacin or other nutrients, these decisions raise many interesting ethical issues.[7]

Here is a comparison between vitamin B$_3$ and Vioxx as it applies to arthritis:

TABLE SHOWING COMPARISON BETWEEN B$_3$ AND VIOXX FOR TREATMENT OF ARTHRITIS		
	VITAMIN B$_3$	VIOXX
What is it?	Vitamin	Drug
Cures?	Yes	No
Relieves pain?	Yes	Yes
Negative side effects?	Minor, not toxic	Major
Positive side effects?	Many	None
Toxic?	No	Yes
Causes deaths?	No	Many
Costly?	Cheap	Expensive
Patented?	No	Yes

Psaty and Kronmal examined pooled data from two studies that showed a significant increase in deaths from Vioxx with "overall mortality of 34 deaths among 1,069 rofecoxib patients and 12 deaths among 1,078 placebo patients. These mortality analyses were neither provided to the FDA nor made public in a timely fashion. The data submitted by the sponsor to the FDA in a Safety Update Report in July 2001 used on-treatment analysis methods and reported 29 deaths (2.7%) among 1,067 rofecoxib patients and 17 deaths (1.6%) among 1,075 placebo patients. This on-treatment approach to reporting minimized the appearance of any mortality risk. In December 2001, when the FDA raised safety questions about the submitted safety data, the sponsor did not bring these issues to an institutional review board for review and revealed that there was no data and safety monitoring board for the protocol 078 study. The findings from this case study suggest that additional protections for human research participants, including new approaches for the conduct, oversight, and reporting of industry-sponsored trials, are necessary."[8]

Ross et al. (2008) present a case-study review of industry documents that demonstrates that clinical trial manuscripts related to rofecoxib were authored by sponsor employees, but they often attributed first authorship to academically affiliated investigators who did not always disclose industry financial support. Review manuscripts were often prepared by unacknowledged authors and subsequently attributed authorship to academically affiliated investigators, who often did not disclose industry financial support.[9] (For more on this topic, see Hill, et al., "The ADVANTAGE Seeding Trial" in the For Further Reading section of this book.)

Based on these two reports, an article by DeAngelis and Fonanarosa concluded: "The profession of medicine, in every aspect—clinical, education, and research—has been inundated with profound influence from the pharmaceutical and medical device industries. This has occurred because physicians have allowed it to happen, and it is time to stop."[10] In another hard-hitting report, Taylor summarized these revelations of the drug industry's mode of operation as "Manipulated studies, conflicts of interest and threats to the public confidence in their medical system."[11] It is about time that the public is introduced to what really has traumatized it for so many years. The cost in deaths, disease, and failure to treat adequately has been enormous.

CHAPTER 8

Children's Learning and Behavioral Disorders

ADHD is not a disease; it is a nutritional deficiency.
—LENDON H. SMITH, M.D.

I n an old "Shoe" cartoon strip, an overweight, cigar-smoking "Perfesser" is sitting at a diner counter. He is urged to eat his carrots because it's been shown that they prevent cancer in rats. His response is, "Why would I want to prevent cancer in rats?" Then there is methylphenidate (Ritalin), which has been shown to promote cancer in mice. This drug is cheerfully given to millions of attention deficit hyperactivity disorder (ADHD) children every day. The *Massachusetts News* (November 1, 1999) placed the figure at 4 million. Yet four years before that, the National Institutes of Health Toxicology Study (July, 1995) stated, "There was some evidence of carcinogenic activity of methylphenidate (Ritalin) in male and female B6C3F1 mice based on the occurrence of hepatocellular neoplasms (liver cancer)."[1] This small but demonstrated carcinogenic potential of this commonly-prescribed drug deserves more attention and much more consideration of safer alternatives. Any bets on how many compliant parents have seen, let alone actually read, the full text of Ritalin's other side effects? Fortunately, there appears to be a vastly safer alternative: vitamins, particularly vitamin B_3.

B_3 AND HYPERACTIVITY

Over fifty years ago, niacinamide pioneer William Kaufman, M.D., Ph.D., observed: "Some patients have a response to niacinamide therapy which seems to be the clinical equivalent of 'decreased running' observed in experimental animals. When these animals are deprived experimentally of certain essential nutriments, they display 'excessive running,' or hyperkinesis. When these deficient animals receive the essential nutriments in sufficient amounts for a sufficient period of time, there is exhibited a marked 'decrease in running. . . [A person] in this group may wonder whether or not his vitamin medications contain a sedative. He recalls that before vitamin therapy was instituted, he had a great deal of energy and 'drive,' and considered himself to be a 'very dynamic person.' Analysis of his history indicates that prior to niacinamide therapy he suffered from a type of compulsive impatience, starting many projects which he left unfinished as a new interest distracted him, returning perhaps after a lapse of time to complete the original project. Without realizing it, he was often careless and inefficient in his work, but was 'busy all the time.'"

This report appeared, almost as a side note, on page seventy-three of Kaufman's 1949 book, *The Common Form of Joint Dysfunction*. So accurately does it describe the problems of ADHD children that it is difficult to believe that vitamin B_3 (which never causes cancer) has been so thoroughly ignored for so long.

Kaufman continues: "With vitamin therapy, such a patient becomes unaccustomedly calm, working more efficiently, finishing what he starts, and he loses the feeling that he is constantly driving himself. He has leisure time that he does not know how to use. When he feels tired, he is able to rest, and does not feel impelled to carry on in spite of fatigue. If such a patient can be persuaded to continue with niacinamide therapy, in time he comes to enjoy a sense of well-being, realizing in retrospect that what he thought in the past was a superabundance of energy and vitality was in reality an abnormal 'wound-up' feeling, which was an expression of aniacinamidosis (niacin deficiency)."[2]

Dr. Evan Shute began investigating the use of vitamin E for abruptic plancentae in 1936 and discovered it cured cardiovascular disease. Even before this, Max Gerson, M.D., was treating migraine headaches with vegetable juices, and therein found an effective therapy for various forms of cancer. William Kaufman treated arthritis patients with niacinamide and noticed that it was also an effective remedy for hyperactivity and lack of mental focus. These and other natural healthcare milestones highlight just how dissimilar orthomolecular medicine and drug medicine truly are. While conventional medical authority would promptly admit malnutrition as one cause of cancer, and certainly as a cause of heart disease, there is a profound reluctance to allow that optimum nutrition could be curative of either. With ADHD, orthodox medicine seems unwilling even to admit nutrient deficiency as a causal factor, let alone a curative one.

Parents can change that. Just say no to drugs. Consider nutrition and niacin instead.

Nutrition, Niacin, and Children

How many years does it take for a new way of treating behavior disorders in children to be generally accepted? The answer is forty, according to Abram Hoffer. There are few physicians who have sufficient experience to personally validate such a claim, but Dr. Hoffer could. He pioneered megavitamin research and treatment back in the early 1950s, and, half a century later, has still been largely ignored by the medical profession. In fact, Hoffer had a seventeen-year jump on Pauling; vitamin B$_3$ (niacin or niacinamide) to treat behavioral disorders was first used by Hoffer and his colleague Dr. Humphrey Osmond in 1952. Niacin worked then, and it works now.

I (AWS) knew of a ten-year-old boy who was having considerable school and behavior problems. Interestingly enough, the child was already on physician-prescribed little bits of niacin, with a total daily dose of less than 150 mg. Not a bad beginning, since the RDA for kids is under 20 mg per day. But it wasn't enough to be effective, and the boy was slated for the Ritalin-for-lunch bunch. Dr. Hoffer suggested trying him on 500 mg niacinamide three times daily (1,500 mg total). That's a lot, but niacinamide is a comfortable, flush-free form of vitamin B$_3$. So Mom tried it.

What a difference!

People often ask, "If this treatment is so good, how come my doctor doesn't know about it? How come it is not on the news?" The answer may have more to do with medical politics than with medical science. Consider Dr. Hoffer's views on attention deficit hyperactivity disorder: "The DSM system [Multiaxial Diagnostic System, the standard of the American Psychiatric Association] has little or no relevance to diagnosis. It has no relevance to treatment, either, because no matter which terms are used to classify these children, they are all recommended for treatment with drug therapy" sometimes combined with other non-megavitamin approaches. "If the entire diagnostic scheme were scrapped today, it would make almost no difference to the way these children were treated, or to the outcome of treatment. Nor would their patients feel any better or worse."[3] Statements like these do not exactly endear one to the medical community.

Criticisms and even lawsuits over the hazards of tranquilizers, Ritalin, and related pharmaceuticals are on the rise, but neither court nor controversy can cure your child. "Battered parents" (Hoffer's term) need to know what to do, and now. Saying "no" to drugs also requires saying "yes" to something else. That something else is nutrition, properly employed. For those who say there is insufficient scientific evidence to support megavitamin therapy for children's behavior disorders, we say they haven't been looking hard enough. Hoffer and his colleagues conducted the first double-blind controlled-nutrition trials in psychiatric history in 1952.

I (AH) have seen well over two thousand children under the age of fourteen since 1955.[4] The result of orthomolecular treatment in which vitamin B$_3$ is the main constituent has been very good, without the need to use any medication. In the early days I did on occasion use very small doses of antidepressants for children who were bed wetters. Later I would simply eliminate the foods they were allergic to. Most of the children recovered. Recovery depended more on the cooperation of their parents, who were able to persuade even recalcitrant children that they should take their vitamins. More recently I have seen former child patients who brought their children in.

Here are a few examples to illustrate the results. One of the first was Mary (not her real name), who at age seven had been diagnosed as mentally retarded. This is too harsh a term for modern parents, and to please them, psychiatry adopted other equally erroneous names such as the ADD series of diagnoses. Mary's mother was schizophrenic. Mary could not learn, she was developing behavioral problems, and she was being readied for classes for the retarded. I was asked to see her by a friend. At that time I had little experience in treating children. I could not see anything wrong with her and had to accept her parent's observations. I started Mary on niacinamide, 1 gram after each of three meals. Two years later she was no better, and I saw her again. Not knowing what else to do, I suggested patience and that they should continue the supplementation. She recovered the third year. Mary completed university on the Deans List, became a music teacher, married, raised her family, and has since retired. A small amount of a vitamin turned her life around.

Instead of being a burden to herself and her family, she became a productive and normal member of society.

In 1960, a physician phoned me, very worried about his twelve-year-old son, who was schizophrenic. His psychiatrist had advised him that he would never recover, and to lock him up and forget about him. Following my advice, he obtained niacin, but the psychiatrist refused to give it to him, stating that they had tried it, it had never worked, and it would fry his brain. All lies. So his father began to visit him every day, and while they were walking about the grounds of the hospital, he fed his son jam sandwiches containing niacin. About twelve weeks later his son said, "Daddy, I want to go home." He later became a doctor, and one summer he worked in Professor Linus Pauling's laboratory. A small amount of a vitamin saved his life and family, and converted a tragic outcome into a normal and happy one.

The next patient was a seven-year-old boy, who would race into his parent's bedroom at night. The boy told me that during the night, a huge vulture would fly through the closed door and that he ran into his parents' bedroom to save them from the vulture. I started him on a slow-release niacin, 1 gram taken after each of three meals. He recovered. He called me many decades later to touch base. He was a successful professional and still remembered that hallucination, as he now called it. He had forgotten why he ran into his parents' bedroom.

Another patient was a teenage boy, who came for treatment in 1973. He is now a professor at a major university. And recently a man diagnosed as schizophrenic in 1976 at age sixteen came by to check whether he was still on the correct orthomolecular program. In the meantime he had married, had two children both doing well, and was working full time. He also tried to leave time for his art, which he enjoyed. I wonder how many orthodox psychiatrists can describe similar recoveries using only drugs.

The treatment of children has become even more toxic over the past five years. It suddenly became fashionable to diagnose children, even babies, as bipolar.[5] Over one million children in the United States are being treated with adult atypical antipsychotic drugs. These drugs are poisoning huge numbers of unfortunate psychotic patients worldwide with the following side effects: diseases such as metabolic syndrome (diabetes, high blood cholesterol, high blood triglycerides), increased complications from cardiovascular pathology, neurological diseases such as tardive dyskinesia, deterioration of brain function, tranquilizer psychosis, permanent social incapacity, suicide, homicide, serial killers, broken marriages and homes, homelessness, addictions to drugs and alcohol, more people in prison, more people on welfare, more postsurgical delirious reactions of the aged on statins after surgery.

Why would anyone allow these toxic poisons to be inflicted on any population, child or adult?

Nutrition and Children with Severe Mental Challenges

There are literally hundreds of thousands of books and articles that illustrate the benefits of treating and preventing disease with high doses of nutrients. A few of the most spectacular of these publications describe the work of Dr. Ruth Flinn Harrell.[6,7] Initially, Dr. Harrell used nutrient-rich foods and later, as they entered the marketplace, high doses of vitamins to treat children who had lost major parts of their brains to cancer and then to surgery. Beyond this, she treated Down syndrome and mentally challenged children in a similar manner. Her successes were spectacular. Most of these children, after nutritional treatment, returned to take their places in the normal school system.[8] Improvements in IQ in some patients were in the 50–60 point range. One such child, who at the age of seven had never spoken a word and still wore diapers, learned to read and write at his appropriate elementary school levels, ride a bicycle and skateboard, and play team ball games. After forty days of high dose nutrients, his IQ rose from the 25 to 30 point range to 90. Dr. Harrell and her research team used nutritional dosages that were greatly in excess of those recommended for adults. (See the table below for details.) Her "super feeding" regimen for learning-disabled children included much larger doses of vitamins than other researchers are inclined to use: over 100 times the adult (not child) RDA for riboflavin; 37 times the RDA for niacin (given as niacinamide); 40 times the RDA for vitamin E; and 150 times the RDA for thiamine. Supplemental minerals and natural desiccated thyroid were also given. Harrell's team achieved results that were statistically significant, some with confidence levels so high that there was less than one chance in a thousand that the results were due to chance. Simply stated, Ruth Harrell found IQ to be proportional to nutrient dosage. This may simultaneously be the most elementary and also the most controversial mathematical equation in medicine.[9] Ruth

Flinn Harrell's approach yielded smarter, happier children. Her results are sufficiently compelling justification for a therapeutic trial of orthomolecular supplementation for every learning-impaired child. Anyone wishing to learn more about Dr. Harrell's research is advised to read Dr. Saul's 2004 article in the *Journal of Orthomolecular Medicine*, "The Pioneering Work of Ruth Flinn Harrell: Champion of Children" and also the description of her research in Dr. Hugh Desaix Riordan's book *Medical Mavericks, Volume 3*. The article by Dr. Harrell and colleagues, published in the *Proceedings of the National Academy of Science USA* in 1981, is also is well worth reading.

DR. RUTH HARRELL'S NUTRIENT DOSES FOR LEARNING-DISABLED CHILDREN	
NUTRIENT	DOSE
Vitamin A palmitate	15,000 IU
Vitamin D (cholecalciferol)	300 IU
Thiamin	300 mg
Riboflavin	200 mg
Niacinamide	750 mg
Calcium pantothenate	490 mg
Pyridoxine hydrochloride	350 mg
Cobalamin	1,000 mcg
Folic acid	400 mcg
Vitamin C (ascorbic acid)	1,500 mg
Vitamin E (d-alpha-tocopheryl succinate)	600 IU
Magnesium (oxide)	300 mg
Calcium (carbonate)	400 mg
Zinc (oxide)	30mg
Manganese (gluconate)	3mg
Copper (gluconate)	1.75mg
Iron (ferrous fumarate)	7.5mg
Calcium phosphate	37.5 mg
Iodide (KI)	0.15 mg

Fetal Alcohol Syndrome

Drinking alcohol while pregnant may create children who are learning impaired and have behavioral problems. This is known as fetal alcohol syndrome or FAS. Treatment is entirely psychosocial. Drugs commonly given to children to treat FAS, like Ritalin and Dexedrine, have been of no value. They are not even palliative. Two girls with FAS were given excellent psychosocial and nutritional care, but recovered only after supplements were added. This shows that the damage done by the alcohol is not permanent and can be corrected by giving these children the right doses of the B vitamins, especially B_3. It also suggests that had their mothers been taking more of the B vitamins, they would have given birth to normal babies free of FAS.

The B vitamin thiamine is also extremely valuable in correcting problems associated with alcohol poisoning, as seen in Wernicke-Korsakoff syndrome. There is, of course, a point of high-dose alcohol damage that can be irreversible. The best cure is prevention, and the best prevention is to stop drinking.

Hoffer and Foster wrote:

> The sins of one's parents are often visited upon their children and this applies particularly to fetal alcohol syndrome. These unfortunate, innocent children have not sinned. The metabolic derangement caused by the mother's use of alcohol during pregnancy surely is also present in the fetus and they are left with a major problem for which there appears to be no simple effective treatment. Hoffer treated several of these children with a multivitamin program with success. One of the main ones is vitamin B_3. The last two patients treated have shown convincingly that this is the right approach and of course will not do any harm. Here are their stories:
>
> LR, born in May 1994 and seen September 2004 had been diagnosed with fetal alcohol syndrome. Her great aunt took her for care. She had been neglected, later counseled but she continued to have major difficulty in focusing and she would have to be asked the same question over and over again. She learned slowly and she suffered mood swings. She was hypervigilant and physically aggressive toward her younger sister. Dexedrine made her much worse and caused severe nightmares and visual illusions and Ritalin, which was not as toxic as the Dexedrine, did not have any therapeutic effect.

Her aunt placed her on a dairy-free program, which was followed by major improvement. Hoffer added niacin 100 mg after each meal, ascorbic acid 500 mg after each meal, the essential fatty acids and a multivitamin complex. She did not like the niacin flush and her B_3 was changed to inositol niacinate (no-flush niacin) 500 mg three times daily. When seen ten months later she was almost normal. But because she had lost so much valuable learning experience her aunt planned to have her go to a special school where she would be able to receive more attention from her teachers. She was cheerful, relaxed and in Dr. Hoffer's opinion was well on the way to complete recovery."[10]

By October 2008 she was a very good "A" student. Her personality was pleasant, helpful, and considerate. There was no question that she was normal and a delight to her family.

Her younger sister was born in March 2001. She was examined at the same time as her sister and appeared to be normal. It seemed likely that fetal alcohol syndrome might express itself later on. She was started on a similar program and when she was last seen she too showed major improvement and was normal.

Ieraci and Herrera found that injecting mouse pups with alcohol caused death of brain cells and behavioral changes. However, this damage was prevented when the pups were subsequently injected with nicotinamide. They recommended that "it is worth pursuing nicotinamide as a possible treatment for preventing FAS in situations where a pregnant woman is unable to stop drinking entirely."[11]

NUTRITION AND BEHAVIOR

As discussed earlier, exceptionally high doses of nutrients can result in major positive changes in the behavior of children who have suffered significant brain trauma and in children with Down syndrome and other serious mental challenges. At lower dosages, it is apparent that such substances also can significantly improve antisocial behavior.

In May 2004, the Dutch Ministry of Justice provided the British Home Office with an evaluation of literature linking antisocial behavior and diet.[12] It argued that this novel approach was very cost effective, allowing both an improvement of services and an 18 percent cost savings.[13] Strangely enough, the research in question originated in the United Kingdom. In 2003, Gesch and colleagues from the University Laboratory of Physiology, University of Oxford, had reported on the results of a randomized, placebo-controlled trial.[14] This study was designed to discover if adequate vitamin, mineral, and essential fatty acid intake reduced antisocial behavior in 231 young adult prisoners, inmates at HMYOI (Her Majesty's Young Offenders Institution) Aylesbury. For nine months, these "volunteers" were given either a placebo or capsules containing the generally accepted daily requirements of vitamins, minerals, and essential fatty acids. In addition, the subsequent number of proven offenses committed by each participant was recorded. When the trial code was broken, it was discovered that those prisoners who had received additional nutrients had committed an average of 26.3 percent fewer offenses than those in the inmate placebo group. The reduction of more serious offenses, involving violence, in the nutritionally enriched group was 37 percent. Both of these declines in antisocial behavior in the supplement group are statistically significant.

The realization that nutrition has a major impact on how humans behave is not new. As pointed out by Jack Challem[15] in the 1970s, Bill Walsh, a scientist at Argonne National Laboratory was also working as a volunteer at Illinois' Stateville Prison. His experiences led him to compare mineral levels in the hair of twenty-four pairs of brothers. In each case, one brother was a well-behaved member of society, while the other was a "boy from hell." The results were amazing. The hair analyses showed that well-behaved males had normal mineral levels, but the imprisoned delinquents all showed one of two abnormal patterns. "Boys from hell" had either very high copper and very low zinc, sodium, and potassium levels in their hair or very low zinc and copper and very high sodium and potassium. In addition, the delinquents also had lead and cadmium levels that were three times greater than those of their well-behaved siblings.

Walsh subsequently found the same minerals abnormalities in a group of 192 adults, 50 percent of whom were incarcerated and the other 50 percent law abiding. He also discovered that the two distinct, abnormal mineral and toxin levels in the hair of prisoners were linked to specific behavioral traits. Inmates with very high copper and very low zinc, sodium, and potassium levels in their hair had repeated uncontrollable temper losses. After their bursts of anger, such prisoners felt remorse for their actions. Prisoners with very low levels of copper and zinc combined with very high levels of sodium and potassium were always complaining, were mean, cruel, and defiant, and were never remorseful. They were typical sociopaths. Walsh eventually conducted hair mineral analysis on 28 mass murderers and serial killers. Each fell into one of the two abnormal mineral patterns. Although it is not entirely clear why some people have such unusual mineral levels in their hair and apparent associated antisocial behavior, Walsh believed that it reflected poor metallothionein function (metallothionein is a cysteine-based protein that transports metals such as copper, zinc, and cadmium in the body) that in infancy increased the probability of mercury, lead, and cadmium poisoning. Whether or not this interesting hypothesis is correct, it is clear that mineral and vitamin levels in the human body have a profound influence on human behavior, and this is still largely ignored.

CHAPTER 9

Mental Illness

For schizophrenics, the natural recovery rate is 50 percent.
With orthomolecular medicine, the recovery rate is 90 percent.
With drugs, it is 10 percent. If you use just drugs,
you won't get well.
—ABRAM HOFFER, M.D., PH.D.

The United States Patent Office delayed issuing a patent on the Wright brothers' airplane for three years because it broke accepted scientific principles.[1] This is actually true. And so is this: Vitamin B_3, niacin, is scientifically proven to be effective against psychosis, and yet the medical profession has delayed endorsing it. Not for three years, but for nearly sixty.

In 1952, our late coauthor Abram Hoffer, M.D., Ph.D., had just completed his psychiatry residency. What's more, he had proven, with the very first double-blind, placebo-controlled studies in the history of psychiatry, that vitamin B_3 could cure schizophrenia. You would think that psychiatrists everywhere would have beaten a path to Saskatchewan to replicate the findings of this young Director of Psychiatric Research and his colleague, Humphrey Osmond, M.D.

You'd think so.

In modern psychiatry, niacin and schizophrenia are both terms that have been closeted away out of sight. And patients, tranquilized into submission or Prozac-ed into La-La Land, are often sitting idly at home or wandering the streets. Either way, it is highly doubtful that they will get much in the way of a daily vitamin intake. Those in institutions fare little better nutritionally. For everyone "knows" that vitamins do not cure "real" diseases.

For over half a century, Dr. Hoffer has dissented. His central point has been this: Illness, including mental illness, is not caused by drug deficiency. But much illness, especially mental illness, can be caused by a vitamin deficiency. This makes sense and has stood up to clinical trial again and again.

NUTRITION, NIACIN, AND MENTAL HEALTH

I (AWS) personally should have first become aware of a food-brain connection during the all-night, cookie-fired mah-jongg marathons that I indulged in all too regularly while attending Australian National University. Though arguably I was somewhat less than psychotic, my mind was nevertheless pretty whacked out on sugar, junk food, and adrenalin by 3:00 AM. My mood was destroyed; my mind agitated; I was unable to sleep, sit still, or smile. Of course, I never entertained even the thought of a nutrition connection. For we've all been carefully taught that drugs cure illness, not diet.

And certainly not vitamin supplements!

But the truth will come out eventually. Three years later, I first saw niacin work on somebody else. He was a bona fide, properly diagnosed, utterly incurable, state-hospitalized schizophrenic patient. I did not see niacin work in the hospital, of course. The only vitamins given there are those your body can filter out of your tray of sweetened, overcooked, overprocessed food. No, the patient was a fellow whose parents were desperate enough try anything, even nutrition. Perhaps this was because their son was so unmanageably violent that he was kicked out of the asylum and sent to live with them. On a good day, his mom and dad somehow got him to take 3,000 mg of niacin and 10,000 mg of vitamin C. Formally a hyperactive insomniac, he responded by sleeping for eighteen hours the first night, and became surprisingly normal within days. I'd seen him before, and I saw him after. I'd talked to his parents during the whole process. It was an astounding improvement.

Sometime afterward, I tried niacin to see if it would help my own touch of sleeplessness. I found it worked nicely, and it only took a little to do so, perhaps 100 mg at most. Any more and I would experience a warm flush. But then I found that when I ate junk food or sugar in quantity, I could hold 500 mg or more without flushing a bit. And when I took all that niacin, instead of flipping out, I was calm. Dr. Hoffer[2] has explained why this is so:

1. Generally speaking, the more ill you are, the more niacin you can hold without flushing. In other words, if you need it, you physiologically soak up a lot of niacin. Where does it all go? Well, a good bit of it goes into making nicotinamide adenine dinucleotide, or NAD. NAD is just about the most important coenzyme in your body. It is made from niacin, as its name implies.

2. Niacin also works in your body as if it were an antihistamine. Many persons showing psychotic behavior suffer from cerebral allergies. They need more niacin in order to cope with eating inappropriate foods. They also need to stop eating those inappropriate foods, chief among them the ones they may crave the most: junk food and sugar.

3. There is a chemical found in quantity in the bodies of schizophrenic persons. It is an indole called adrenochrome. Adrenochrome (which is oxidized adrenalin) has an almost LSD-like effect on the body. That might well explain their behavior. Niacin serves to reduce the body's production of this toxic material.

I have taught nutritional biochemistry to high school, undergraduate, and chiropractic students. To most, it is not an especially gripping subject. But when even a basic working knowledge of niacin chemistry can profoundly change psychotic patients for the better, it becomes very interesting very quickly.

Dr. Hoffer treated thousands and thousands of such patients for over half a century. Medical fads come and go. But what we see today is what he saw all along: that even severely mentally ill people get well on vitamin B_3.

The Physiological Role of Niacin

David Horrobin followed my (AH) observation that schizophrenic patients did not flush as much by developing a flush skin test, which has been amply corroborated. This increased researchers' interest in niacin receptors in the skin and elsewhere. Later the G protein-coupled niacin-responsive receptors HM74A and HM74 were identified. HM74A has a high affinity for niacin. Miller and Delay[3] found that the protein for HM74A was decreased in schizophrenic brains compared with bipolar and normal controls. They suggest that "The possibility a deficiency in the high-affinity niacin receptor is a core feature of many individuals with schizophrenia provides a basis for research into more potent receptor agonists and therapies that might significantly increase expression of the fully functional protein." This can be an explanation of the therapeutic value of niacin, which we discovered in 1952, and could account for the fact that so much is needed. Miller and Delay wrote: "In conclusion, one important implication of the data presented here is that the early clinical studies by Abram Hoffer reporting in a notable degree of success through treatment of unmedicated patients with niacin, but inconsistently, replicated in follow-up work by others, should now be reevaluated in the context of the limitations imposed by a deficient receptor. . . . The possibility that a deficiency in the high affinity niacin receptors is a core feature of many individuals with schizophrenia provides a basis for research into more potent receptor agonists and therapists that might significantly increase expression of the fully-functional protein."

In 1973, I wrote in *Orthomolecular Psychiatry,* edited by Hawkins and Pauling: "It is possible and, if the views presented here are reasonably close to the truth, even highly probable, that the genetic errors which underlies the schizophrenias is an enzymatic block between tryptophan and NAD."[4] Later, Hoffer and Foster wrote, "Niacin is not a true vitamin in the strictest sense of the term since it can be produced in the body from the amino acid tryptophan. Nevertheless, the synthesis of niacin from tryptophan is a very inefficient process and 60 milligrams (mg) of the amino acid are necessary to provide 1 mg of niacin. This process also involves vitamins B_1, B_2, and B_6. If these are in short supply, the synthesis of vitamin B_3 will be even less efficient." It must also be remembered that tryptophan itself is not usually very readily available in diet; especially in those eating high levels of maize.

It is clear, therefore, that humans have the ability to synthesize niacin, but this process is ineffective and is probably in evolutionary decline. Of course, vitamin B_3 is also available from many foods. If the diet contained enough of this vitamin to supply bodily requirements, there would be no need to convert tryptophan to niacin. This would liberate energy for other uses and free up tryptophan for the production of serotonin, a major neurotransmitter. It is argued that humanity has been depending more and more on vitamin B_3 derived from diet. However, recently, niacin has become less available from food. As a result, subclinical pellagra and other niacin deficiency disorders are becoming very widespread.

In a private communication to AH, Miller wrote:

> A study of postmortem brain tissue was undertaken in this laboratory to quantify the protein for the high affinity niacin receptor. Although peripheral tissue bears more relationship to the blunted cutaneous flush response, it is obviously brain function that is most relevant to the schizophrenic condition. A comparison of postmortem brain samples derived from controls and schizophrenia patients revealed that the protein for the high affinity niacin receptor was significantly decreased in the schizophrenia group.
>
> This raised the possibility of a genetic defect that would impair the amount of protein synthesized and thereby result in a compensatory upregulation of the mRNA transcript for the niacin receptor. Subsequent genetic association studies in a large cohort have confirmed that a polymorphism in the niacin receptor HM74 gene is associated with schizophrenia and bipolar disorder (Miller et al., submitted). Furthermore, the identified polymorphism affects gene expression in a manner consistent with the gene-expression difference seen between cases and controls.[5]

There is a great deal of evidence to support this argument. Some 50 percent of the population of the developed world seems to suffer from disorders or diseases that respond beneficially to niacin or niacinamide supplementation. This figure is probably an underestimate, as detailed in Chapter 3. Indeed, the authors believe that the addition of 100 mg of niacinamide to the public diet would enormously reduce human suffering and have a major impact on the unnecessary escalation of health care costs. This additional niacinamide would probably nearly return the daily dietary intake to that of centuries ago, before the advent of food processing and widespread artificial fertilizer use. This suggested strategy is not new. During the Second World War, the United States government mandated the enrichment of flour with niacinamide. It is clear, however, that current dietary levels are still too low. Increasing the intake of niacinamide would not have any known risks, since it is not addictive or a narcotic, nor is it a euphoriant or an analgesic. In short, a small investment in niacinamide would provide huge economic and social benefits to society with no known associated risks. It must be recognized, however, that some people would require far more vitamin B_3 than others, either because of pre-existing diseases and disorders, or as a result of their genetic inheritances.

"The question remains, 'Why would a genetic aberration, lowing niacin production in the body that could result in so many diseases or disorders become so widespread amongst the human population?' Perhaps the answer can be obtained by studying sickle-cell anemia. Roughly one out of every 400 Black Americans develops sickle-cell anemia. In those with this chronic hereditary disease, many of their red blood cells form rigid crescent or sickle shapes that cannot pass through capillaries. Affected children often die during adolescence of strokes, heart disease, and infections. Sickle-cell anemia also causes sufferers painful, unpredictable health crises. Those children that survive are underweight and slow to mature. How is it that a genetic, highly damaging disease can be so widespread amongst the Black population in the USA? What's in it for Darwin? Or more correctly asked, what is the evolutionary advantage that this mutation gives to Blacks that makes its obvious disadvantages worthwhile? After all, as McElroy and Townsend point out, 'It is only the phenotypic characteristics that give some advantage of degree of Darwinian fitness that are subject to selective action.'"[6]

So what is going on? Vitamin B3 (niacin or niacinamide) is involved in almost all the oxidation and reduction reactions in the body. Tryptophan is processed in the body into a number of very important substances. The overall pathway leading from tryptophan to NAD (nicotinamide adenine dinucleotide) and NADH (NAD plus hydrogen), the active antipellagra coenzymes, is not very efficient. It converts less than 2 percent of tryptophan into these enormously important substances. A major pathway for conversion is the kynurenine pathway. This enzyme is more active in schizophrenic brains, and this can account for the decrease in the formation of B3 by diverting more of the tryptophan into this pathway instead of into B3.[7]

A block between tryptophan and NAD might provide an evolutionary advantage, as long as dietary (exogenous) vitamin B3 was high. It now appears that there are several possible genetic pathways. And among these we must include those needed to maintain NAD levels in the body, those that permit the production of excess amounts of adrenochrome, and those that prevent an optimum supply of the antioxidants. Modern views of the genes possibly involved are discussed by Foster and Hoffer in their reports. A deficiency of the NAD$\longleftrightarrow$NADH system may be one of the most important causes. There are many triggers but most of them can be overcome with the use of adequate supplementation with vitamin B_3, which leads to an increased amount of NAD in the body.

Indoleamine 2,3-dioxygenase (IDO) is necessary for the degradation of tryptophan into B_3. We do not know if IDO activity is higher in schizophrenics. There is probably a higher-than-normal expression of the nicotinic acid G-protein coupled receptor.[8,9,10]

The discovery of nicotinic acid (niacin) receptors in the brain may help us understand why schizophrenic patients become so easily addicted to nicotine and find it so difficult to stop. I have been aware of this for decades and have been puzzled by it.[11] Nicotine, the poison, might be involved in the same biochemical reactions as niacin.[12]

There are probably several relationships between smoking (nicotine) and schizophrenia. I have advised clients who have schizophrenia not to stop smoking until they showed substantial progress on the orthomolecular program. If nicotine does attach to the nicotinic acid receptors it may also act as a therapeutic imitator of niacin. If nicotine were not so toxic, it might be a very valuable treatment. But its toxicity overwhelms its benefits, and patients should discontinue its use as soon as it becomes possible. If they do not get well, they will not stop smoking. Luckily, schizophrenic patients do not get cancer of the lungs to the same extent as the rest of the population.[13] Nicotine may be considered a very toxic analogue of niacin. It is not surprising that taking niacin makes it easier for smokers to stop their habit.[14]

Psychiatric Disorders Need Niacin in Particular

To treat schizophrenia and schizoaffective disorder, the main emphasis should be on vitamin B_3. I have successfully treated over 5,000 patients this way.

Schizophrenia is not a multivitamin deficiency disease. It is pellagra, a vitamin B_3 dependency, and it will not be treated successfully, no matter how many dozens of vitamin pills are given, if these patients are not given the correct doses of this vitamin. You can give pellagrans every known nutrient, but if you do not give them B_3 they will still remain pellagrans.

Nowhere in many reports have I suggested that schizophrenia was a multivitamin deficiency disease. I have always maintained that it was a *B_3 dependency disease*, and that large and sometimes very large doses were needed. A few patients I did not see took up to 60 grams each day on their own without any side effects. One must use this important vitamin, and it is easy to deal with the side effects that may be troublesome but hardly ever serious, and do not kill. Does anyone ever read those reports? In the past few months three patients consulted with me. They had been treated for up to ten months by orthomolecular psychiatrists and had not responded to treatment. But when I looked over the treatments they were on, I was astonished that I could not find any B₃ on their lists. They were taking large numbers of pills containing nearly every known nutrient, but they were schizophrenic and not suffering from a multivitamin deficiency disease, so they were not healed. In one case a young man, who was making substantial and steady progress, was taken off his B₃ and started on some other natural products and promptly relapsed. On resuming his B₃ intake, he continued to recover and has now been well several years.

I can not believe that doctors could have failed so miserably to realize that while all the vitamins are helpful in restoring health, recovery will not occur if the schizophrenic patient (pellagrin) is not given the B₃ they require. A patient with pellagra can be given tons of vitamins, but they will not recover until the right amount of B₃ is added. And in most patients I have seen who failed to get well, most of the other vitamins they were taking were not needed, as they are available in food. In other words, they were forced to buy exorbitant amounts of pills they did not need. If your patients have scurvy, give them ascorbic acid, not niacin. If they are schizophrenic, give them vitamin B₃—but in the right doses.

Schizophrenia and pellagra differ in that pellagra needs small doses of vitamin B₃ in most cases and schizophrenia needs large doses in most cases. As discussed in Chapter 3, pellagra is a deficiency and schizophrenia is a dependency.

From our first publications in 1954, Osmond and I emphasized that large doses of B₃ are needed to treat schizophrenia. Unfortunately, the vasodilatation (flush) caused by niacin when it is first taken has given niacin a bad name. Even today most doctors are more fearful of this vitamin, which kills no one, than they are of the major atypical antipsychotics, which kill many. The flush is a minor problem when niacin is used by doctors who know what they are doing. I had hoped that the results I have published—with hundreds of case histories, confirmed by every physician who used the same protocols—would have made other doctors comfortable with niacin by now. But unfortunately this has not happened.

I foresee a major problem in getting physicians to accept this treatment if a large number of patients are only treated with multivitamins and do not get enough B_3. The establishment will believe they are correct in concluding that there is no connection between schizophrenia and the use of B_3, and this valuable treatment will be set back another forty years. I do not think I will be sent to prison, but I fear for the schizophrenic patients all over who will have lost their chance for healing. Instead, they will be given modern equivalents of mercury, alum, nitre (and, of course, ever more tranquilizers) to correct the fanciful imbalances of "humors in the brain" (the neurotransmitters).

THE MAIN PSYCHOTIC DISORDERS

Of the $150 billion the United States spends per year on psychiatric care, the lion's share goes for drugs to treat psychotic disorders. Niacin can be useful to many of these patients. Niacin, given along with conventional drug therapy, reduces the amount of medication needed and reduces medication side effects. Niacin greatly reduces costs and increases treatment success.

The psychotic disorders are differentiated into primary groups, which can be identified by their characteristics.

The Schizophrenias

Schizophrenic disorders are characterized by perceptual changes (hallucinations) and thought disorder (delusions). These are pellagra syndromes, including Huntington's disease, some Parkinsonism patients, schizoaffective patients, and LSD induced psychosis. I consider these conditions variants of pellagra. Schizoaffective patients have mood swings, and during their manic states will also have schizophrenic symptoms. These pellagra variants are responsive to vitamin B_3 when adequate doses are used. They will not respond to small doses or to other nutrients. They are B_3 *dependent* conditions, and should not be considered as deficiency diseases. Too many clinicians have ignored this and have tried to treat their patients with a multiplicity of nutrients but without using enough B_3. They therefore have not seen the therapeutic results that occur when the correct dose of this vitamin is used.

Patients with Parkinson's disease tend to develop psychosis and this is more probable when they take L-dopa, which in the brain can be converted into dopachrome. Niacin protects them from the psychosis and coenzyme Q_{10} (CoQ_{10}) protects against neurological changes such as tremor.

Both niacin and niacinamide are antidotes to the LSD reaction.[15] If 100 mg of niacin is given intravenously to a person under the influence of LSD, most of the reaction will be gone in a few minutes. Many years back, when we were routinely using psychedelic treatment for alcoholics, we would terminate the experience with either IV niacin or oral niacin (500 mg three times daily) if it lasted too long or if it became too unpleasant for the subjects.

Schizoaffective Disorder

Schizoaffective patients should be treated as if they were schizophrenic. Lewis and Pietrowski[16] found that half of a large series of manic-depressive (bipolar) patients, followed up during subsequent hospitalizations, were clearly schizophrenic by their final diagnosis. This important study has been overlooked or ignored by modern psychiatry, which tends to call anyone with a mood swing "bipolar" no matter how schizophrenic they are during their manic phase. I have seen the same change in diagnosis with repeated admissions.

I have written about the orthomolecular treatment of the schizophrenias over the past fifty years. A large literature of clinical studies is available in standard journals and in the *Journal of Orthomolecular Medicine*, beginning with our very first double-blind studies.

Letter from a Patient

I'm writing to thank you for changing my life. You may remember that I was in despair: I thought I'd have to quit my job, and most days were pretty miserable for me. Niacin changed everything. It enables me to enjoy my teaching once more, to be able to relate to the students and anyone else, to think and communicate clearly, and just to be a "normal" person. Like you said, it's not perfect, but the improvement has been incredibly great. I also take the other vitamins and follow the other suggestions you made to me, but the niacin is at the heart of it all. If only I had called you years ago. But the niacin sure helped when things were at their worst. Thank you again.

Bipolar Disorder

Bipolar disorder is characterized by a series of mood swings, which swing from mania to depression and normal in between. Most of the time, there are no perceptual symptoms or thought disorder. The cycle varies tremendously from once a month to once every few years. Modern drugs distort the typical cycle and in many cases convert depression into mania.

When normal or depressed, bipolar patients do not suffer the typical schizophrenic symptoms, but during manic episodes they may often hear voices and see visions, which clear as the mania clears. We therefore have at least two types of bipolar: those who never have any schizophrenic symptoms and those who do when they are manic. How, then, are we to differentiate the two types? Psychiatry got around this by giving those who suffer from schizophrenic episodes both diagnoses: they are called schizoaffective.

These types also respond differently to orthomolecular therapy. Non-schizophrenic bipolar patients need mood-stabilizing treatment, while the schizoaffective patients need this treatment plus treatment for the schizophrenic component of their disease. I find that schizoaffective patients are much easier to treat than bipolar or schizophrenic patients.

Diagnosis can be very difficult for these patients, and often it depends more on the orientation of the diagnostician than on the disease itself. The diagnosis, schizophrenia, is so dismal and carries such a poor prognosis that many physicians prefer not to consider it. If their patients have mood swings, minor or major, they will call them bipolar. A large proportion of the schizophrenic patients referred to me were originally called bipolar, and their perceptual changes had either not been elicited or were ignored. In a major recent study, Weiser et al.[17] found that nearly 30 percent of a schizophrenic population had been diagnosed with affective disorder during adolescence compared with only 7 percent of the general population. This confirmed what I have been seeing for the past fifty years.

Niacin treatment is similar for all psychotic patients. Many years ago I did not consider that vitamin B_3 would be useful in treating bipolar patients. I was still in my "establishment" stage, from which I have recovered. Over the years I have become more and more aware of the importance of niacin for bipolar patients. Several years ago a middle-aged woman consulted with me. She had been diagnosed as schizoaffective, with two enforced admissions to the hospital. Each time she was force-treated with drugs, which she stopped taking when she was discharged. But after her last discharge she started to take niacin, an astonishing 30 grams in the morning and again in the evening. By the time I saw her six months later, she was normal. She told me she would rather take 120 pills of 500 mg niacin daily than any of the awful drugs she had been given in the hospital. Very, very few patients can take so much niacin without developing severe nausea and vomiting.

Delirium, Including Delirium Tremens

Dr. Humphry Osmond and I developed a treatment protocol for alcoholics in delirium tremens (DTs) or in a predeleriod state. On admission, they were given niacin (500 mg I.V. and 3,000 mg oral) and ascorbic acid (2,000 mg). On the first day, they received niacin (3,000 mg) after each of three meals, the same amount of vitamin C, and a sedative, if needed. This was to be continued until they were free of the delirium. The results were very dramatic. In most cases, delirium tremens and acute alcoholic intoxications respond well within twenty-four hours. For this purpose, it is as good as the tranquilizers that were commonly used at the time, but it has the added advantage that there is no sedation. The patient remains more alert and, after a few hours, is cooperative. There are no toxic complications. Our studies in Saskatchewan corroborated Dr. Gould's observations in England. These doses were much larger than the usual recommended daily doses.

I have routinely given patients niacin to reverse delirium or to protect them from developing perceptual disturbances that predominate in deliria. These deliriod states, called DTs, are common in alcoholics and in other drug-induced toxic conditions. Niacin will be very useful in protecting statin-induced delirium after surgery. Redelmeier et al.[18] found that patients are at greater risk for developing postoperative delirium if they were on statins. Mercantonio[19] concluded that the use of statins increased the incidence by 30 percent, even though the study his conclusion was based upon underestimated the risk. However, being too cautious, they did not recommend stopping the statins. There is no need to use the statins at any time, since niacin is much superior to any individual statin or combination of statins. It is the only compound that effectively increases high-density cholesterol levels in blood, which is the most important risk factor for vascular disease when it is too low. If patients were taking niacin instead of the statins, they would also be protected against postsurgical deliria.

Post-Electroconvulsive Confusion

In 1952 a very unhappy man and very confused woman came to me for help. I could get no information from her, but her husband told me she had been very depressed and had been committed to the mental hospital where she had been given a series of electroconvulsive therapy (ECT) treatments. She was discharged home but had been totally confused for the next month. She displayed a typical organic confusional state, as if she were developing Alzheimer's disease. I had never seen a patient with this reaction to ECT and really did not know what to do, but I had read of niacin's use for confusional states in the 1940s and was certain it would do no harm. I started her on 1 gram taken three times daily after meals, and mailed her a supply from my office as 500 mg tablets were not available in stores. When I saw her again one month later, I saw an entirely different couple. He was cheerful and she had regained her previous normal personality. There was no evidence of confusion.

At the sixth meeting of the Saskatchewan Committee on Schizophrenia Research (June 11–12, 1953) I reported, "Often the underlying psychosis is banished by ECT and instead is replaced by a mental picture including memory loss, confusion, and aggressivity. EEG [electroencephalogram] records show some neuropsychological pathology; Lehmann first reported that these respond well to niacin. We have not run a series to further test this but plan to do so. Further, it may be successful in preventing the confusion following epileptic convulsions." This was the beginning of my conviction that niacin must always be given with ECT, and this conviction has become stronger every year. Since then, I would never give any patients ECT without niacin. I consider that giving ECT without niacin should be looked upon as malpractice.

I have not needed to use ECT for many years, but there have been a few times when I recommended to patients that they should receive it from their psychiatrist. I think the art of giving ECT with minimum discomfort and minimum memory loss and maximum therapeutic effect is being lost. It causes much less harm than antipsychotic drugs.

CHAPTER 10

Cardiovascular Disease

Niacin is really it. Nothing else available is that effective.
—STEVEN E. NISSEN, M.D., PRESIDENT OF
THE AMERICAN COLLEGE OF CARDIOLOGY

It is well established that niacin helps reduce harmful cholesterol levels in the bloodstream. Niacin is one of the best substances for elevating high density lipoprotein cholesterol (the "good" cholesterol), and niacin provides other valuable cardiovascular benefits as well.

But you'd never know this from the headlines. A recent study has been frequently trumpeted to imply that niacin does not work, and that it is somehow detrimental. That, to put it scientifically, is a lot of baloney. Specifically, the researchers reported that the drug simvastatin worked better than simvastatin with Niaspan. Niaspan, an extended-release form of niacin, is alleged to have caused about a 1 percent increase in cardiovascular events. The drug somehow evaded suspicion, and blame was attached to the vitamin. That in itself is questionable. What's more, in this study there was no examination of Niaspan alone. There was also no consideration at all of immediate-release, plain old regular niacin. Regular niacin works just fine, and safely.[1]

FROM BLEEDING GUMS TO CORONARY DISEASE

In 1954, it was impossible to predict or even to think that my (AH) bleeding gums would one day, thirty-one years later, lead to additional useful life to people with coronary disease related to cholesterol and lipid metabolism. That year, malocclusion of my teeth had broken down the ability of my gum tissue to repair itself. My incorrect bite caused too much wear

115

and tear on tooth sockets, and my gums began to bleed. No amount of vitamin C and no amount of dental repair helped. Eventually I reconciled myself to the idea I would soon have all my teeth extracted.

But at this time I had been treating schizophrenia, senility, and a few other diseases with niacin, and I began also to take this vitamin myself— 1 gram after each meal, for a total of three grams per day. I did so because I wanted to experience the flush that comes when one first takes niacin as well as its gradual waning with continued use so I could discuss these reactions more knowledgeably with my patients. There was also a legal issue. Most doctors' defense against malpractice suits is that they were doing what other similar physicians would do in similar circumstances. If I were sued (I have never been) because of unusual discomfort or adverse effects from niacin, I would not be able to use that defense since only a handful of physicians had ever used such large quantities of niacin. I concluded that if the unlikely occurred and I was charged with malpractice, one of my defenses would be that I had tried it myself for at least three months without suffering serious consequences. I must admit I did not discuss this with a litigation lawyer. My reasons were therefore both practical and paranoid—but I had no intention of treating myself or my bleeding gums.

Two weeks after I had started taking niacin, my gums were normal. I was brushing my teeth one morning and suddenly awakened in surprise that there was no bleeding whatever! A few days later, my dentist confirmed that my gums were no longer swollen. I still have most of my teeth. Eventually I reasoned that the niacin had restored the ability of my gum tissue to repair itself faster than I could damage it by chewing with my crooked teeth.

A few months later I was approached by Rudolf Altschul, Chairman, Department of Anatomy, College of Medicine, University of Saskatchewan. I had been one of his students when he taught neurohistology. Professor Altschul had discovered how to produce arteriosclerosis in rabbits: he fed them a cake baked by his wife, Anna, which was rich in egg yolks. Rabbits fed cooked egg yolk promptly developed hypercholesterolemia and later arteriosclerotic lesions on their coronary vessels.[2] Altschul had also discovered that irradiating these hypercholesterolemic rabbits with ultraviolet light decreased their cholesterol levels. He wanted to extend this research by irradiating human subjects, but not one internist in Saskatoon would allow him access to their patients. (People who bake in the southern sunshine may wonder why this "dangerous" treatment received such a negative response.) Professor Altschul thus approached me. As Director of Psychiatric Research, Department of Health, Saskatchewan, I had access to several thousand patients in our two mental hospitals. I agreed to this research provided that Dr. Humphry Osmond, Superintendent of the Saskatchewan Hospital at Weyburn, also agreed. The treatment was innocuous, would not cost us anything, and would help us create more of an investigative attitude among our clinical staff. But before we started, I requested that Professor Altschul meet with our clinical staff and present his ideas to them.

A few weeks later he came to Regina by train, and I drove him to Weyburn in my car to meet Dr. Osmond and his staff. On the way down and back we discussed our work. He gave me an interesting review of how he saw the problem of arteriosclerosis, which he considered to be a disease of the intima, the inner lining of the blood vessels. He hypothesized that the intima had lost its ability to repair itself quickly enough. As soon as I heard this I thought of my bleeding gums and of my own repair hypothesis. I then told him of my recent experience. I asked him if he would be willing to test niacin, which might have antiarteriosclerotic power if it had the same effect on the intima as it had had on my bleeding gums. Professor Altschul was intrigued, and agreed to look at the idea if he could get some niacin. I promptly sent him one pound of pure, crystalline niacin from a supply I had received earlier, courtesy of Merck and Company.

One evening about three months later, I received a call from Professor Altschul who began to shout, "It works! It works!" Then he told me he had given niacin to his hyperlipidemic rabbits and within a few days, their cholesterol levels were back to normal. He had discovered the first hypocholesterolemic substance. Drug companies were spending millions to find such a compound.

But did it also work in humans? The next day I approached Dr. J. Stephen, Pathologist at the General Hospital, Regina. I was a biochemical consultant to him. I outlined what had been done and wanted his help in some human experiments. I assured him niacin was safe and we would only need to give a few grams to patients. He promptly agreed. He said he would order his technicians to draw blood for cholesterol assay from a large variety of patients, would then given them niacin, and would follow this with another cholesterol assay. I suggested we discuss this plan with the patients' physicians, but Dr. Stephen laughed and said they did not know what went on in the hospital, and that to contact each one would probably make the study impossible. A few weeks later the data poured in: niacin also lowered cholesterol levels in people. The greater the initial or baseline level, the greater the decrease.

We published our results. This report initiated the studies which eventually proved that niacin increases longevity.[3] This was not a double-blind study, but patients did not know what they were getting or why they were getting it. This type of impromptu research is now impossible with ethics committees, informed consent, and so on. Thirty years ago, only the integrity of physicians protected patients against experimental harm.

At the same time we were examining the effect of niacin on cholesterol levels, Russian scientists were also measuring the effect of vitamins on blood lipids. However, they used very little niacin and found no significant decreases.[4]

The finding that niacin lowered cholesterol was soon confirmed by Parsons and his colleagues in a number of studies at the Mayo Clinic, which launched niacin on its way as a hypocholesterolemic substance. Since then it has been found to be a normalizing agent in that it elevates high density lipoprotein cholesterol, decreases low density and very low density lipoprotein cholesterol, and lowers triglycerides. Grundy and his colleagues found that niacin lowered cholesterol by 22 percent and triglycerides by 52 percent and wrote, "To our knowledge, no other single agent has such potential for lowering both cholesterol and triglycerides."[5]

The Coronary Study

The only reason for being concerned about elevated cholesterol levels is that it is associated with increased risk of developing coronary disease. The association between cholesterol levels in the diet and coronary disease is not nearly as high, even though the overall diet is a main factor. The kind of diet generally recommended by orthomolecular physicians will tend to keep cholesterol levels down in most people. This diet can be described as a high fiber, sugar-free diet rich in complex polysaccharides such as vegetables and whole grains.

Once it became possible to lower cholesterol levels with no alteration in diet, it became possible to test the hypothesis that lowering cholesterol levels would decrease the risk of developing coronary disease. Dr. E. Boyle, then working with the National Institute of Health, Washington, D.C., quickly became interested in niacin. He began to follow a series of patients using 3 grams (3,000 milligrams/mg) of niacin per day. He reported his conclusions in a document prepared for physicians in Alcoholics Anonymous by Bill W. in 1968.[6] In this report, Boyle reported that he had kept 160 coronary patients on niacin for ten years. Only six died, against a statistical expectation that 62 would have died with conventional care. He stated, "From the strictly medical viewpoint, I believe all patients taking niacin would survive longer and enjoy life much more."[7]

His prediction came true when the National Coronary Drug Study was recently evaluated by Canner. But Boyle's data spoke for itself. Continuous use of niacin will decrease mortality and prolong life. Perhaps Boyle's study was one of the reasons the Coronary Drug Project was started in 1966. Dr. Boyle was an advisor to this study, which was designed to assess the long-term efficacy and safety of five compounds in 8,341 men, ages thirty to sixty-four, who had suffered a myocardial infarction (heart attack) at least three months before entering the study.

The National Heart and Lung Institute supported this study. It was conducted at fifty-three clinical centers in twenty-six American states and was designed to measure the efficacy of several lipid-lowering drugs and determine whether lowering cholesterol levels would be beneficial for patients with previous mycardial infarctions. Niacin, two dosage strengths of estrogens, Clofibrate, dextrothyroxine, and a placebo were tested.

Eighteen months after the study began, the higher-dose estrogen group in the study was discontinued because of an excess of new non-fatal myocardial infarctions that occurred among patients using this drug compared to those on the placebo. The thyroxine group was stopped for the same reason for patients with frequent ectopic ventricular beats. After thirty-six months, dextrothyroxin was discontinued for the rest of the group, again because myocardial infarctions were increased compared to the placebo. After fifty-six months, the low-dose estrogen group study was stopped. There had been no significant benefit to compensate for the increased incidence of pulmonary embolism and thrombophlebitis and increased mortality from cancer. Eventually only the niacin, Clofibrate, and placebo groups were continued until the study was completed.

Canner's Follow-up Study

Dr. Paul L. Canner, Chief Statistician, Maryland Medical Research Institute, Baltimore, examined the data that came out of the Coronary Drug Project Research Group trial. About 8,000 men were still alive at the end of the treatment trial in 1975. Canner's study began in 1981, to determine if the two estrogen regimens and the dextrothyroxine regimen had caused any long-term effects. As described above, the high-dose estrogen had been discontinued because it increased nonfatal myocardial infarctions, low-dose estrogen increased cancer deaths, and dextrothyroxine increased total mortality compared to placebo, Clofibrate, and niacin. None of the subjects continued to take the drugs after 1975.

The 1985 follow-up study showed no significant differences in mortality between the treatment groups that had been discontinued and the placebo or Clofibrate groups. However, to the investigator's surprise, the niacin group fared much better. The cumulative percentage of deaths for all causes was 58.4 percent, 56.8 percent, 55.9 percent, 56.9 percent, and 50.6 percent respectively for low-dose estrogens, high-dose estrogens, Clofibrate, dextrothyroxine, and placebo.

The mortality in the niacin group was 11 percent lower than in the placebo group. The mortality benefit from niacin was present in each major category or cause of death: coronary, other cardiovascular, cancer, and others. Analysis of life table curves comparing niacin against placebo showed that niacin patients lived two years longer. With an average follow-up of fourteen years, there were seventy fewer deaths in the niacin group than would have been expected from the mortality rate in the placebo group. Patients with cholesterol levels higher than 240 mg per 100 dL benefited more than those with lower levels.

What is surprising is that the niacin benefit carried on for such a long period, even after no more was being taken. In fact, the benefit increased with the number of years followed up. It is highly probable the results would have been much better if patients had not stopped taking niacin in 1975. Thus, Boyle's patients who remained on niacin for ten years and received individual attention had a *90 percent decrease in mortality.* In the huge coronary study, this type of individual attention was not possible for the majority of patients. Many patients dropped out because of the niacin flush and may have been persuaded to remain in the study if they had been given more individual attention. This level of attention is very hard to do in a large-scale clinical study of this type. Dr. Boyle mentioned this as one of the defects in the Coronary Drug Study in his discussions with me. I would conclude that the proper use of niacin for similar patients should decrease mortality somewhere between 11 and 90 percent after a ten-year follow-up, with the longevity increasing, especially in patients with elevated cholesterol levels.

In 1985 National Institute of Health released a conference statement, "Lowering Blood Cholesterol to Prevent Heart Disease,"[8] based on the conclusions reached by a consensus development conference in 1984 on lowering blood cholesterol to prevent heart disease. It reports that heart disease kills 550,000 Americans each year, and 5.4 million are ill. Total costs of heart disease (at that time) were $60 billion per year. Main risk factors for heart disease include cigarette smoking, high blood pressure, and high blood cholesterol. The NIH recommended that the first step in treatment should be dietary, and their recommendations are met by the orthomolecular diet. When diet alone is not adequate, drugs should be used. Bile-acid sequestrants and niacin were favored while the main commercial drug, Clofibrate, was not recommended, "because it is not effective in most individuals with a high blood cholesterol level but normal triglyceride level. Moreover, an excess of overall mortality was reported in the World Health Organization trial of this drug."

Since niacin is effective only in megavitamin doses, 3,000 mg (1,000 mg three times per day), NIH was at last promoting megavitamin therapy. The National Institute of Health asked that their conference statement be "posted, duplicated, and distributed to interested staff." Since every doctor has patients with high blood cholesterol levels, they should all be interested. One reason why they may not be is because NIH seems to have cooled its enthusiasm, such as it ever was, for high-dose vitamin therapy. If you go to the NIH website to read the pro-niacin conference statement, there is a prominent, red-letter editorial warning that:

> This statement is more than five years old and is provided solely for historical purposes. Due to the cumulative nature of medical research, new knowledge has inevitably accumulated in this subject area in the time since the statement was initially prepared. Thus some of the material is likely to be out of date, and at worst simply wrong. For reliable, current information on this and other health topics, we recommend consulting the National Institutes of Health's MedlinePlus.[9]

We question the neutrality of such commentary. NIH's MedlinePlus and Medline/PubMed online indexes are selective filters and a long way from comprehensive.[10]

The Effect of Niacin When Combined with Other Drugs That Lower Cholesterol

Familial hypercholesterolemia is an inherited disease in which plasma cholesterol levels are very high. Illingworth and colleagues described a study of a series of thirteen patients treated with Colestipol, 10 grams twice daily and later 15 grams twice daily. Their cholesterol levels ranged from 345 to 524 with triglycerides from 70 to 232. When this drug plus diet treatment did not decrease cholesterol levels below 270, they were given niacin, starting with 250 mg three times daily and increasing it every two to four weeks until 3 to 8 grams per day was reached. To reduce the flush, patients took aspirin (120 to 180 mg) with each dose for four to six weeks. Researchers found no abnormal liver function test results with this dose of niacin. This combination of drugs normalized blood cholesterol and lipid levels. The authors concluded, "In most patients with heterozygous familial hypercholesterolemia, combined drug therapy with a bile acid sequestrant and nicotinic acid (niacin) results in a normal or near normal lipid profile. Long-term use of such a regimen affords the potential for preventing, or even reversing, the premature development of atherosclerosis that occurs so frequently in this group of patients."[11]

At about the same time Kane and his colleagues reported similar results on a larger series of fifty patients. They also studied the combined effect of Colestipol and Clofibrate. Abnormalities of liver function only occurred when the dose of niacin increased rapidly. Patients took 2.5 grams per day the first month, 5.0 grams per day the second month, and 7.5 grams per day the third month and thereafter. Blood sugar went up a little (from 115 to 120 mg) in a few patients and uric acid levels exceeded 8 mg percent in six patients. None developed gout. All other tests were normal. They concluded, "The remarkable ability of the combination of Colestipol and niacin to lower circulating levels of LDL . . . suggests that this combination is the most likely available regimen to alter the course of atherosclerosis."[12] The combination of Colestipol and Clofibrate was not as effective. For the first time it was seen that it is possible to extend the life span of patients with familial hypercholesterolemia.

How Reliable is Medline Plus?

Both Medline and MedlinePlus have a history of bias in favor of pharmaceutical medicine and against vitamin therapy. Medline/PubMed is used primarily by doctors and academics. MedlinePlus is aimed at the general public. Both are taxpayer funded. Medline censorship has been the subject of several articles:

Saul, A. W. "NLM censors nutritional research: Medline is biased, and taxpayers pay for it." *Orthomolecular Medicine News Service* (Jan 15, 2010).

Saul, A. W., S. Hickey. "Medline obsolescence." *Journal of Orthomolecular Medicine,* 22(4) (2007): 171–174. Editorial.

Saul, A. W. "Medline bias." *Townsend Letter for Doctors and Patients* 277/278 (Aug-Sep 2006): 122–123. Editorial

Saul, A. W. "Medline bias: update." *Journal of Orthomolecular Medicine* 21(2) (2006): 67. Editorial.

Saul, A. W. "Medline bias. *Journal of Orthomolecular Medicine.* 20(1) (2005): 10–16. Editorial

As to the objectivity of MedlinePlus, you can check for yourself at www.nlm.nih.gov/medlineplus/. A MedlinePlus search (June 2011) for "orthomolecular" brought up exactly four results. Two were from the American Cancer Society, one from the MD Anderson Cancer Center, and one from the American Academy of Pediatrics. None of the articles had more than a very brief mention of orthomolecular medicine, and none of the comments were positive. *There were no MedlinePlus search responses whatsoever to any orthomolecular book, article, or website.* Medline Plus is paid for by your tax dollars. Is information selectivity something you wish to fund?

Fortunately, niacin does not decrease cholesterol to dangerously low levels. Cheraskin and Ringsdorf[13] reviewed some of the evidence that links low cholesterol levels to an increased incidence of cancer and greater mortality in general. Ueshima, Lida and Komachi[14] found a negative correlation between low cholesterol levels and cerebral vascular disorders. Mortality increased for levels under 160 mg. Further research found that the hypocholesterolemic action of niacin was related to the activity of the autonomic nervous system. Niacin also lowered cholesterol levels of schizophrenic patients, but to a different degree than in normal patients.[15–17]

Why Does Niacin Lower Cholesterol?

It is important to note that although all forms of vitamin B_3 are anti-pellagra and are almost equally effective in treating schizophrenia, arthritis, and a number of other diseases, only niacin (not niacinamide) lowers cholesterol. The no-flush niacin ester, inositol hexaniacinate, is also effective in lowering cholesterol and triglyceride levels.[18] Niacin also differs from niacinamide in that it causes a flush, while niacinamide has no vasodilation activity in 99 percent of the people who take it. For reasons unknown, about 1 in 100 persons who take niacinamide do flush. They must be able to convert niacinamide to niacin in their bodies at a very rapid pace.

In 1983 I (AH) suggested that niacin lowers cholesterol because it releases histamine and glycosaminoglycans. Niacinamide does not do this. A histamine-glycosaminoglycan-histaminase system had also been found to be involved in lipid absorption and redistribution in an earlier study by Mahadoo, Jaques, and Wright in 1981.[19] Boyle had found that niacin increased basophil leukocyte count; these cells store heparin as well as histamine. He suggested that the improvement caused by niacin is much greater than can be explained by its effect on cholesterol, and that improvement may be due to release of histamine and also to a reduction in intravascular sludging of blood cells.

It is possible the beneficial effect of niacin is not due to the cholesterol effect but is due to a more basic mechanism. Are elevated cholesterol levels and arteriosclerosis both the end result of a more basic metabolic disturbance that is still not identified? If it were entirely an effect arising from lowered cholesterol levels, why did Clofibrate not have the same beneficial effect? An enumeration of some other properties of niacin may one day lead to this basic metabolic fault. Niacin has a rapid anti-sludging effect. Sludged blood is present when the red blood cells clump together. The clumps are not able to traverse the capillaries as well as regular cells, as they must pass through in single file. This means that tissues will not receive their quota of red blood cells and will suffer anoxemia. Niacin changes the properties of the red cell surface membrane so that they do not stick to each other. Tissues are then able to get the blood they need. Niacin acts very quickly and increases healing, as it did with my gums. Perhaps it has a similar effect on the damaged intima of blood vessels. Niacin appears to directly help reduce inflammation.

In the past few years, adrenalin, via its aminochrome derivatives, has been implicated in coronary disease. If this becomes well established, it provides another explanation for niacin's beneficial effect on heart disease. In a series of reports Beamish and his coworkers showed that myocardial tissue takes up adrenalin, which is converted into adrenochrome and it is the adrenochrome that causes fibrillation and heart muscle damage.

Under severe stress as in shock or after an injection of adrenalin, a large amount of adrenalin is found in the blood and is absorbed by heart tissue. Severe stress is thus a factor whether or not arteriosclerosis is present, but it is likely an arteriosclerotic heart can not cope with stress as well as a healthy heart. Fibrillation would increase demand for oxygen, which could not be met by a heart whose coronary vessels are compromised.

Niacin protects tissues against the toxic effect of adrenochrome, in vivo. It reverses the EEG changes induced by intravenous adrenochrome given to epileptics,[20] and also reverses the psychological changes.[21] In synapses (gaps between nerve cells), nicotinamide adenine dinucleotide (NAD) is essential for maintaining noradrenalin and adrenalin in a reduced state. These catecholamines lose one electron to form oxidized amine. In the presence of NAD, this compound is reduced back to its original catecholamine. If there is a deficiency of NAD, the oxidized adrenalin (or noradrenalin) loses another electron to form adrenochrome (or noradrenochrome). This change is irreversible. The adrenochrome is a synaptic blocking agent, as is LSD. Thus niacin, which maintains NAD levels, decreases the formation of adrenochrome. It is likely this also takes place in the heart, and if it does, it would protect heart muscles from the toxic effect of adrenochrome and from fibrillation and tissue necrosis. None of the other substances known to lower cholesterol levels are known to have this protective effect. Niacin thus has an advantage in lowering cholesterol and decreasing frequency of fibrillation and tissue damage.

Niacin as a Treatment for Acute Coronary Disease

A number of practitioners have used niacin clinically, as soon as possible after an acute event. These include C. E. Goldsborough, who used both niacin and niacinamide in this way between 1946 and 1960.[22] Patients with coronary thrombosis were given niacin, 50 mg by injection subcutaneously and 100 mg sublingually. As the niacin flush developed, the pain and shock of the coronary subsided. Another injection was given if the pain recurred when the flush faded, but if the pain was not severe another oral dose was used. The patient was given 100 mg three times daily after that. If the flush was excessive, niacinamide was used instead.

Goldsborough treated sixty patients during this period, twenty-four with acute infarction and the rest with angina. From the twenty-four patients, six died. Four of the angina patients also had intermittent claudication, which was relieved by the treatment. Two had pulmonary embolism and also responded favorably.

Niacin should be used before and after every coronary bypass surgery. Inkeless and Eisenberg reviewed the evidence related to coronary artery bypass surgery and lipid levels in 1981.[23] There is still no consensus that this surgery increases survival. In most cases the quality of life is enhanced, and 75 percent get partial or complete relief of angina. I believe a major problem not resolved by cardiovascular surgery is how to halt the arteriosclerotic process. Inkeles and Eisenberg report that autogenous vein grafts implanted in the arterial circuit are more susceptible to arteriosclerosis than arteries. In an anatomic study of ninety-nine saphenous vein grafts from fifty-five patients who survived thirteen to twenty-six months, arteriosclerosis was found in 78 percent of hyperlipidernic patients (elevated blood lipid, especially cholesterol). Aortic coronary-bypass grafting accelerates the occlusive process in native blood vessels.

If patients were routinely placed on the proper diet and, if necessary, niacin long before they developed any coronary problems, most if not all coronary bypass operations could be avoided. If every patient requiring this operation were placed on the proper diet and niacin following surgery, the progress of arteriosclerosis would be markedly decreased. Then surgeons would be able to show a marked increase in useful longevity.

Niacin increases longevity and decreases mortality in patients who have suffered one myocardial infarction. *The Medical Tribune* properly expressed the reaction of early investigators by heading their April 24, 1985 report, "A Surprise Link to Longevity: It's Nicotinic Acid." More recently, niacin has been demonstrated to reduce injury to the brain after strokes.[24]

Elevated cholesterol levels are associated with increased risk of developing coronary disease. In addition to niacin, we also recommend a high fiber, sugar-free diet high in vegetables and whole grains. However, with adequately high doses of niacin, it is possible to lower cholesterol levels even with no alteration in diet. Continuous use of niacin will decrease mortality and prolong life. Incidentally, abnormally low cholesterol is not a niacin effect. Niacin does not decrease cholesterol to dangerously low levels.

In 2007, the *New York Times* reported that inexpensive vitamin B_3, niacin, "can increase HDL as much as 35 percent when taken in high doses, usually about 2,000 milligrams per day. It also lowers LDL, . . .

Statins versus Niacin

A reader writes:

"Almost every day I read or see an article on statins and how good they are for you, and how more people should be taking them. I wonder. I was put on Zocor to lower cholesterol and after some time I experienced pain in shoulders. I was told to take warm showers. But no, I wanted to stop taking Zocor. So I was put on Pravachol, and after a time every joint (and I mean *every* joint) in my body was in agony. I was told I wasn't getting younger, and the doctor wanted to prescribe pain pills. I said no. I refused to take Pravachol any more. Lo and behold, in a matter of months gradually my joints stopped hurting. For the most part I have returned to my old self. However I did lose muscle tone to a great degree. When I was going through this, I know my doctor thought, 'This one is paranoid,' but I know what I felt. Can you please tell me more about statins?"

If Pravachol sounds like a street near the Kremlin and Zocor sounds like a Klingon, read on. Dr. Hoffer says:

"I would love to see a double-blind, controlled study comparing niacin against any one of the modern statins to be run at least ten years. It would win the battle hands down. And it can be combined with the statins if this is necessary. Diet by itself is relatively ineffective, difficult to follow, and according to Parsons not very practical as it is so difficult to alter people's ways of eating. I agree.

"In his book, *Cholesterol Control Without Diet: The Niacin Solution,* Dr. Parsons reviews the role of the statins and the drug companies that got them approved and placed upon the market. I think this is an important section. And it is not a pretty picture. If your doctor tells you that you have a cholesterol problem, or if you suspect that you might have it, be sure and talk to him about niacin rather than take the statins, and refer him to this excellent book. It will answer all his questions and reassure him that niacin is the right one. You will be better for having done so."

(and) triglycerides as much as 50 percent."[25] The *Times* quoted Steven E. Nissen, M.D., president of the American College of Cardiology, as saying: "Niacin is really it. Nothing else available is that effective."

Niacin was first used to successfully lower serum cholesterol in 1955. Since then, placebo-controlled studies have confirmed that niacin prevents second heart attacks, and niacin also reduced strokes. One study showed that after fifteen years, men taking niacin had an 11 percent lower death rate. Although a warm "flush" is a common side effect of niacin, the vitamin is safer than any drug.

Recently, the non-statin drug Zetia (ezetimibe) was seen to be greatly inferior to niacin in controlled drug trials. Niacin stomped Zetia (a multibillion-dollar drug) so badly they had to stop the clinical trials for the benefit of the patients.[26]

So, for decades, it has been established that niacin not only is the best single substance we know for reversing all the pathological lipid findings in patients with cardiovascular problems, it is the only one. It decreases total cholesterol levels because it decreases the low-density cholesterol, it increases high-density cholesterol, lowers triglyceride levels, lowers lipoprotein(a), and lowers C reactive protein (CRP) levels. CRP is a measure of oxidative stress. None of all the other substances used widely, such as the statins, can even come close to niacin's ability to improve these numbers. In spite of billion-dollar efforts to develop a patentable product with the same beneficial properties as niacin, all efforts have ended in failure, including some deaths. Niacin decreased deaths by 11 percent compared to placebo, according to the Coronary Drug Study described earlier in this chapter. It increased life by two years in middle-aged men who has already suffered at least one coronary. That huge study was the direct outcome of our original finding that niacin lowered total cholesterol and the subsequent confirmation of that finding by studies at the Mayo Clinic.

Our national patent system, which places profit as the only important objective, not the health of its clients, is largely responsible for the fact that these studies have been largely ignored. Governments have allowed Big Pharma to get away with this. It is not surprising that I (AH) have seen many patients given statins, which are not effective and cause serious side effects, when they should have been on niacin. It does take medical skill to prescribe niacin properly. Parsons stated that "One must know niacin in order to use it." Too few physicians have developed this skill. They have not been encouraged by their medical training and have been mislead by overwhelming drug advertising.

It is odd that Big Pharma scientists are not able to understand Roger Williams' argument. To visualize the complexity of reactions in the cell, Williams compared the cell to an orchestra. Each essential nutrient is like one member of that orchestra. A superb symphonic performance is a function of the quality of the musicians, a good conductor, and everyone reading the same music. These criteria are what the public demands. However, suppose during the performance the solo violinist faints. The conductor believes the show must go on, and calls upon the lead drummer to replace the violinist. At this point we will no longer hear a symphony—it will be a cacophony. Recently, in real life, young Kuerti, a conductor, discovered that the pianist for that evening's performance was not able to appear. He called on his father Anton Kuerti, who was at the concert. The symphony was superb. But there is only one Anton Kuerti. In the cells of the body each nutrient has been selected by evolution to be like an Anton Kuerti. If thiamine is removed from the cell only another Kuerti, thiamine, can replace it. It must be replaced and until this is done, the cell will not perform. It will eventually die if the replacement doesn't arrive. Giving a patient a xenobiotic to replace what is missing is like replacing the violinist or pianist with the drummer. It would be like replacing Anton Kuerti with me. The orthomolecular law is that xenobiotics can not replace missing orthomolecular substances. The drug companies are wasting our money, looking for something they will never find.

CHAPTER 11

Other Clinical Conditions That Respond to Niacin

*The person who says it cannot be done
should not interrupt the person doing it.*
—CHINESE PROVERB

I t is hard to justify denying a patient a therapeutic trial with a vitamin. Open-minded, inquisitive physicians never have. The observations, insights, dedication (and often just plain courage) of nutritionally-minded doctors are worthy of our continued appreciation today, a time when some say there is little value in "anecdotal" physician reports and case studies. Medical drug dogma is out of date. Inadequate nutrition, an old problem that has failed to go away, should be addressed first. Doing so will prevent much illness. For existing disease conditions, physicians should begin a therapeutic trial of specific nutrients such as niacin. It is up to each person to insist that their doctor does so. True, this is not always easy. To strengthen both your interest and your resolve, this chapter provides an overview of niacin's many specific clinical uses.

Aging

In April 2008, Miss Kaku Yamanaka died in Japan. She was 113 years old. The oldest person alive in the world at that time was Miss Edith Parker, Indiana, age 114. In Canada, Miss Mary MacIsaac, age 112, died on March 10, 2006. She was Saskatchewan's oldest person, second-oldest in Canada and nineteenth-oldest in the world. Her son believes that she was the oldest in Canada. But Miss MacIsaac differed significantly from the others. She had been taking niacin for forty years before she died. She had cross-country skied until 110 and was photographed playing a piano duet with her great-grandson just before she died. She was weaker, but her mind was clear when she died after a brief illness. She credited the niacin and perhaps she was correct, because niacin does have remarkable antiaging and life-extending properties.

In a large-scale double-blind controlled trial comparing niacin against other substances including a popular cholesterol-lowering drug Atromid, estrogens, thyroid, and placebo, only niacin decreased the death rate. It decreased it by 11 percent and increased longevity by two years. The cohort (group of individuals sharing a characteristic) tested were men who had at least one coronary and who were followed for fifteen years.[1]

This does not mean that everyone taking niacin will live as well and as long. But the evidence is persuasive. I (AH) truthfully tell my clients that if they will take niacin, one of the side benefits will be that they will feel better and live longer.

We have already referred to one of my female patients who lived to age 112. In December 2004, I received the following note from her son:

> "There is one person older in Canada, but only our entry has all her wits about her and can walk. I kidded my sister that General Foods have asked her to recommend their product, and asked her what should be the fee. Seriously, she has always said that she followed the Hoffer program. There is a three-page spread on her in a Saskatchewan paper showing her skiing, rafting, horseback riding etc."

In this brief section on aging, I will review the highlights of this evidence. There is growing support for the idea that with proper nutrition and the use of vitamins, people will live longer. Ames,[2,3] in two stimulating reports suggests that people can live longer by "tuning up their metabolism." By this he means that by adding nutrients to their diets, including niacin, in amounts larger than the RDAs (Recommended Dietary Allowances), many diseases will be treated better, the incidence of cancer will decrease, and aging will be slowed. According to Gutierrez[4,] Bruce Ames, discoverer of the Ames test for mutation and cancer-causing chemicals, concluded that a modern high-calorie, nutrient-deficient diet forces the body into a crisis mode. This is beneficial for short term but harmful for long term, and leads to disease, including cancer. According to recent health surveys, 93 percent of the population failed to meet even the inadequate RDA standards for nutrition.

Linus Pauling, molecular biologist and Nobel Prize winner, stated that these insufficient health standards helped maintain the state of poor health we find in the general population.[5]

This is not surprising, since niacin protects the heart and vascular system and the brain by inhibiting the deposition of plaque in the arteries. It is the gold standard of compounds that lower total cholesterol levels in that it elevates high density cholesterol levels, lowers triglycerides and lipoprotein(a) [Lp(a)], and has anti-inflammatory properties. This has been known for a very long time, although it is not widely appreciated or utilized by the medical profession. The Women's Health Study found that higher blood levels of HDL cholesterol in women is associated with better cognitive functioning.[6] This is another unexpected way by which niacin can help stave off dementia. Of all the cholesterol-lowering compounds, only niacin increases HDL significantly.

Modern studies have revealed additional antiaging properties of niacin that work by direct action on a cellular level. To summarize a few studies in this area: Christoph Westphal and his fellow researchers concluded from their review of the literature that "Sirtuins are anti-aging proteins that have therapeutic potential for a range of diseases of aging, including metabolic disorders, neurodegenerative disorders, cancer, and cardiovascular disease."[7] Sirtuins are NAD-dependent protein decarboxylases related to life extension. Since NAD [nicotinamide adenine dinucleotide] is the active coenzyme made from niacin or niacinamide, this vitamin is important. Kaneko and colleagues confirmed that niacinamide protects against Wallerian degeneration in a 2006 study.[8] Wallerian degeneration follows local damage to the axon of nerve cells. This is a significant component of multiple sclerosis, discussed later in this chapter. Sasaki and his colleagues concluded, on the basis of their studies, that stimulating the NAD pathway may be useful in preventing or delaying axonal degeneration.[9] Yang and his colleagues summarized their work as follows: "A major cause of cell death caused by genotoxic stress is thought to be due to the depletion of NAD from the nucleus and the cytoplasm."[10] Since major causes of death are vascular damage and neurone destruction, it shouldn't be surprising that a substance inhibiting all these toxic events will have antiaging properties.

Indeed, evidence is accumulating that niacin helps recovery of the damaged brain. For example, after experimental strokes in animals, Yang and coworkers found that nicotinamide could rescue viable but injured nerve cells within the ischemic area. Early injection of nicotinamide reduced the number of necrotic and apoptotic neurons. Later injections were not as effective. In their report Yang and Adams concluded, "Early administration of nicotinamide may be of therapeutic interest in preventing the development of stroke, by rescuing the still viable but injured and partially preventing infarction." They also found that this vitamin decreased the progression of neurodegenerative disease. It prevented learning and memory impairment caused by cerebral oxidative stress. According to these studies nicotinamide works more quickly than niacin, but both are interconvertable and, in my opinion, niacin will have an advantage because it dilates the capillaries.

Brain-damaged patients have responded to niacin treatment. It is likely that "chemo brain"—forgetfulness, confusion, or lack of focus experienced by patients undergoing chemotherapy—can be prevented by niacin in the same way that it protects against radiation- and chemotherapy-induced cancers some time after the initial treatment. As many as one quarter of patients complain of "chemo brain." These changes are subtle but real, according to Dr. Daniel H. S. Silverman.[11,12] Dr. Silverman is the head of the neuronuclear imaging section at the University of California Medical Center, Los Angeles. He studied women who had received chemotherapy five to ten years previously. They compared the brain activity of these women to healthy controls. Chemo patients had reduced rates of metabolism in specific regions of the frontal cortex—an area involved in memory recall. The chemo had damaged the brain.

I (AH) have seen very few brain-damaged patients, but the following two cases suggest that niacin can be helpful to brain-damaged individuals. One case was a woman around sixty years old. She had prided herself on her good memory, which was helpful in her study of English literature. I saw her about a year after she had a stroke. She was then anxious, frustrated, and depressed because her memory was no longer reliable as it had been before her stroke. After six months on niacin, 3,000 milligrams (mg) per day, and ascorbic acid, 3,000 mg per day, her memory was so much better that she was able to deal with the residual loss without anxiety and depression. Her doctor had originally advised her that she would have to get used to her memory loss. The second case was a thirty-eight-year-old man. He had been struck on the head by a 1,000-pound object two-and-a-half years before I saw him. He was in a coma for several days and in a hospital for several months. Before his accident, he had been an avid reader and in the ninetieth percentile level for intelligence. Six months later, he could read only at a third-grade level and was in the thirtieth percentile. The last time I saw him after his treatment, he was content with the improvement in his ability to read.

A report in *Annals New York Academy of Science* concluded that niacin-bound chromium (glucose tolerance factor contains niacin and chromium) combined with grape seed extract improved insulin sensitivity, decreased free radical formation, and reduced the symptoms of chronic age-related disorders, including Syndrome X (a combination of insulin resistance, elevated cholesterol or triglycerides, overweight, and/or high blood pressure).

Allergies

Many very serious allergic reactions can be avoided by removing the foods causing the allergy and supplementing the patient with the orthomolecular program, which must include vitamin C and niacin. Miss D.H., born in 1960, was very concerned about pain in her wrists and elbows which had been present for over five years. She also suffered from other allergic and autoimmune symptoms. Her skin was constantly itching, she was overweight, had Raynaud's disease (see below) affecting her fingers, had a leg tremor at night, and had dermatographia, a condition in which lightly scratching your skin causes raised, red lines. She also reacted severely to insect bites. These symptoms were partially relieved by antihistamines, but their side effects (drowsiness, dry mouth and nose, headache, dizziness) were not tolerable.

Allergic reactions began when she was twenty. At the time, testing found her to be allergic to some foods, pets, and many other substances. In mid-2005 she developed hives, which later became so severe she had to be treated in an emergency room. An antihistamine helped but she still suffered from itching on face, arms, and back. In 1996 she was diagnosed with Raynaud's. She continued to suffer from an amazing variety of symptoms. She was under the care of her allergist and several rheumatologists who could not help her when she was advised to consult me. She did so regularly and frequently for advice. Allergies to foods were discussed. She was started on vitamin C, 3,000 milligrams daily, and a small starting amount of niacin, 100 mg three times daily after meals. She continued adjusting her diet and followed the supplemental program. The hives and skin reactions ended, and subsequently her physician reported that she was well. She was still well one year after I first saw her.

For more in-depth discussion of allergies, we suggest you read *Orthomolecular Medicine for Everyone: Megavitamin Therapeutics for Families and Physicians.*[13]

Alcoholism and Other Addictions

Ever since I (AH) met Bill W., the cofounder of Alcoholics Anonymous (AA), I have had a personal interest in the treatment of alcoholism. Bill taught that there were three components to the treatment of alcoholism: spiritual, mental, and medical. AA provided a spiritual home for alcoholics that many could not find elsewhere, and helped them sustain abstinence. But for many AA alone was not enough; not everyone in AA achieved a comfortable sobriety. Bill recognized that the other two components were important. When he heard of our use of niacin for treating alcoholics, he became very enthusiastic about it because niacin gave these unfortunate patients immense relief from their chronic depression and other physical and mental complaints.

Niacin is the most important single treatment for alcoholism, and it is one of the most reliable treatments. And it is safe, much safer than any of the modern psychiatric drugs. Niacin does not work as well when alcoholics are still drinking, but in a few cases it decreased their intake of alcohol until they became abstinent. This conclusion is based on the work my colleagues and I have done since 1953.

I know of many alcoholics who did not want to stop drinking, but did agree to take niacin. Over the years, they were able to reduce their intake gradually until they brought it under control. Some alcoholics can even become social drinkers on a very small scale. I have not found many who could, but I think that if started on the program very early, many more could achieve normalcy. I suspect that treatment centers using these ideas will be made available one day and will be much more successful than the standard treatment today. Current treatment all too often still consists of dumping patients into hospitals and letting them dry out, with severe pain and suffering. When they are discharged, most go right back to the alcohol, the most dangerous and widely-used street drug available without a prescription.

The alcoholic's body needs the proper nutrients in adequate quantities to return to normal metabolic functioning. Bill W. was one of the first alcoholic addicts to benefit from niacin. After his last drink he suffered from decades of anxiety, fatigue, and some depression but was able to make his remarkable contribution, which helped millions of drug addicts. We met at a meeting in New York and became close friends. When I learned of his discomfort, I told him about niacin. He began to take 1 gram after each of three meals, and was normal in two weeks. This was so surprising that he joined me in promoting niacin for members of AA— but first he persuaded thirty of his friends in AA to try it. He found that ten were well in one month, another ten at the end of the second month, and the last ten had not responded at the end of the third month. This was remarkably close to the data I had accumulated. Bill W. then determined to share the good news with doctors in AA. This association appointed a committee of three of their members who studied it and agreed that it was very useful.

Against the opposition of International Headquarters of AA, Bill W. prepared and distributed two communications to physician members of AA. Thousands of copies were distributed. A third communication was distributed after his death. Had Bill W. not died, there is no doubt that the therapeutic use of niacin would be much further advanced than it is today. Andrew Saul and I wrote a book about the treatment of addictions with heavy emphasis on my relationship to Bill W., *The Vitamin Cure for Alcoholism*.[14] (See also Hoffer's *Adventures in Psychiatry*). Several clinics in the United States are treating addicts with orthomolecular methods with great success and up to 80 percent recovery.

The orthomolecular program works best in conjunction with the steps of Alcoholics Anonymous, which we support. As Bill W. realized, niacin helps addicts recover from the anxiety, fatigue, depression, and other discomforts that they usually suffer. This, in our opinion, is the basis for their use of alcohol or drugs. Addicts are not well to begin with. Many alcoholics suffer from increased gastrointestinal permeability.[15] This leads to a decrease in antioxidant status. A daily dose of 100 mg of niacin returns gastrointestinal permeability back to normal when associated with abstinence and a proper diet. In my opinion, a healthy individual will not become an addict. They will drink but in moderation, they may try drugs but eventually decide they do not like the effect. They will therefore not

William Griffin Wilson (1895–1971)

Orthomolecular Medicine Hall of Fame 2006

Bill Wilson is the greatest
social architect of the 20ᵗʰ century.
—ALDOUS HUXLEY

The man who would cofound Alcoholics Anonymous was born to a hard-drinking house-hold in rural Vermont. When he was ten, his parents split up and Bill was raised by his maternal grandparents. He served in the Army in World War I, and although he did not see combat, Bill had more than ample opportunities to drink. In the 1920s, Wilson achieved considerable success as an inside trader on Wall Street, but a combination of drunkenness and the stock market crash drained what was left of his fortune and his capability to enjoy life. Hard knocks, religious experience, and a growing sense that he could best help himself by helping other alcoholics led Bill to create one of the world's most famous introductions: "My name is Bill W., and I'm an alcoholic." Even as Alcoholics Anonymous slowly grew, many of Bill's financial and personal problems endured, most notably depression. Abram Hoffer writes: "I met Bill in New York in 1960. Humphry Osmond and I introduced him to the concept of megavitamin therapy. Bill was very curious about it and began to take niacin, 3,000 mg daily. Within a few weeks the fatigue and depression that had plagued him for years were gone. He gave it to thirty of his close friends in AA. Of the thirty, ten were free of anxiety, tension and depression in one month. Another ten were well in two months. Bill then wrote "The Vitamin B_3 Therapy," and thousands of copies of this extraordinary pamphlet were distributed. As a result, Bill became unpopular with the members of the board of AA International. The medical members, who had been appointed by Bill, "knew" vitamin B_3 could not be as therapeutic as Bill had found it to be. I found it very useful in treating patients who were both alcoholic and schizophrenic.

For further reading:

Hoffer, A. *Vitamin B_3: Niacin and Its Amide.* http://www.doctoryourself.com/hoffer_niacin.html.

Hoffer, A., A. W. Saul. *The Vitamin Cure for Alcoholism.* Laguna Beach, CA: Basic Health Publications, 2008.

Wilson, B. *The vitamin B_3 therapy: The first communication to AA's physicians.* Bedford Hills, NY:/Private publication. 1967.

Wilson, B. *A second communication to AA's physicians.* Bedford Hills, NY:/Private publication. 1968.

become addicted to whatever removes that state of being well. For less healthy persons who do become addicted, they maintain the addiction in order to prevent the withdrawal effects. We do not need fancy or elaborate theories of personality or psychology to account for their addiction. They are all forms of self treatment using drugs. Some are socially acceptable and some are not. AA deals with some of the problems that have been generated by the addiction over years, and helps remove guilt and restore relationships. This is seen even in animals. Low-status monkeys placed in a cage physically close to high status monkeys choose to take cocaine rather than food, if given a choice. High-status animals, under less stress because of their status, are more apt to choose food rather than cocaine.[16,17] Further evidence that alcoholics will conquer their addiction more easily when they become well is the evidence of those alcoholics who refused give up alcohol but agreed to take niacin. We (AH and AWS) have seen that they stop drinking.

Treating addicts is very easy in principle. Simply help them get well, but not by adding still more addicting drugs, even though they may be socially sanctioned and easier to control, like methadone to replace heroin. Niacin is the best substance I know that will do this.

The late Dr. Roger Williams, a chemistry professor at the University of Texas and former president of the American Chemical Society, also wrote extensively on alcoholism. Dr. Williams recommended large doses of vitamins and an amino acid called L-glutamine.[18]

The orthomolecular program is the treatment of choice for alcoholism. The following protocol for alcoholism outlines many of the nutritional factors that have been shown to be very successful on treating this condition.

The Orthomolecular Program for Treatment of Alcoholism

- High doses of vitamin C (as much as 10,000 mg per day or more) to chemically neutralize the toxic breakdown of the products of alcohol metabolism. Vitamin C also increases the liver's ability to reverse the fatty buildup so common in alcoholics.

- Niacin. Dr. Hoffer's most common prescription was 3,000 mg per day, in divided doses.

- B50-complex tablet (50 mg of each of the major B vitamins) several times daily, with meals.

- L-glutamine (2,000 or 3,000 mg). L-glutamine is an amino acid that decreases physiological cravings for alcohol. It is one of the two primary energy providers that burn glycogen to provide fuel to the brain and stimulates many neurofunctions. L-glutamine is naturally produced in the liver and kidneys. Alcohol harms the kidneys and liver, thus supplementation is vital. L-glutamine concurrently reduces cravings for sugar and alcohol.

- Lecithin (2 or 3 tablespoons daily). Lecithin provides inositol and choline, related to the B-complex. It also helps mobilize fats out of the liver.

- Chromium (at least 200 up to 400 mcg chromium polynicotinate daily). Chromium improves carbohydrate metabolism and greatly helps control blood sugar levels. Many, if not most, alcoholics are hypoglycemic.

- A good high-potency multivitamin, multimineral supplement as well, containing magnesium (400 mg) and the antioxidants carotene and vitamin E as d-alpha tocopherol.

We further discuss alcoholism and other addictions in *The Vitamin Cure for Alcoholism*.

Alzheimer's Disease

Increasingly, research evidence makes it more and more plausible that Alzheimer's disease will be treated much more successfully in the near future. But we have to give up the obsessive attempts to find that blockbuster drug that will be the magic pill. Foster, in his recent book *What Really Causes Alzheimer's Disease*,[19] describes its astonishing descent on our aging population. This is already general knowledge, as few families have not seen it attack one of their members.

Alzheimer's disease has traditionally been considered untreatable except by a few drugs, which at best may slow the degenerative process a little. However, there is growing evidence that it can be prevented by the proper use of nutrients.

Specifically, niacin has been demonstrated to have a marvelously protective effect against the development of Alzheimer's disease and cognitive decline. A study of nearly 4,000 people age sixty-five and older showed that those with the lowest niacin intake (an average of 12.6 mg per day) were 80 percent more likely to be diagnosed with Alzheimer's disease than those with the highest intake (22.4 mg per day). The rate of cognitive decline was only about half as much among those with the highest niacin intake when compared to those with the lower intake. Since 22.4 mg of niacin per day achieves such results, it is reasonable to expect that larger doses are likely to be still more effective.[20] Further support for niacin's support of cognitive function was found in research by Green and coworkers, which found that nicotinamide restored cognition in Alzheimer's disease transgenic mice.[21]

We are not suggesting that niacin alone is the answer to Alzheimer's disease. Compelling evidence indicates that early memory loss can be reversed by the ascorbates (vitamin C). Increased risk of Alzheimer's disease has also been linked to low dietary intake of vitamin E and of fish. The elderly should continue to eat well-balanced diets high in calcium, magnesium, selenium, the B vitamins, and essential fatty acids. Foster has argued at length that Alzheimer's disease is caused by an excess of monomeric aluminum in people who are calcium and magnesium deficient.[22]

Alzheimer's disease and other conditions, such as repeated little strokes, are aging factors. A recent report from Rush Institute for Healthy Aging and Center for Disease Control and Prevention, Atlanta, concluded "In this prospective study we observed a protective association of niacin against the development of Alzheimer's Disease and cognitive decline with normal levels of dietary intake, which could have substantial public health implications for disease prevention if confirmed in further research."[23] This study indicates two things: that only a very little niacin goes a long way, and that many of the elderly are not even getting a little.

High HDL protects against dementia, according to the fifteen-year Women's Health Study, in which 4,081 women age sixty-six and older were divided into five quintiles for HDL levels. The highest group had an HDL level of 73 mg/dL and the lowest 36 mg/dL. The women in the highest quintile had five times less change of having cognitive impairment. The only substance that significantly elevates HDL is niacin.

The main B vitamin is niacin, but other nutrients are involved in lowering risk for development of Alzheimer's disease. Other B vitamins, vitamin E, and vitamin C, when taken together, decrease the incidence of Alzheimer's. Dr. Peter Zandi of Johns Hopkins School of Public Health said that "Vitamin E and C may offer protection against Alzheimer's disease when taken together in the higher doses available from individual supplements."[24] These nutrients decreased risk by 78 percent. Essential minerals such as selenium and zinc are also important, as they counteract the accumulation of toxic metals such as aluminum and mercury. Essential fatty acids also play a major role. In short, optimal nutrition will be the most decisive factor in slowing down the ravages of aging.

Niacin may inhibit the development of Alzheimer's disease, but unfortunately I (AH) have not found it helpful in treating the condition once it is established. However, about one-third of all patients diagnosed with Alzheimer's disease will, at autopsy, not show Alzheimer's typical pathological findings. In these cases the clinical syndrome is the same, but the causes are different. I suspect that these patients were more apt to have had a series of small strokes. Niacin will be more helpful for patients such as these. Their cholesterol levels may be an important clue. Alzheimer's patients often have elevated cholesterol levels, suggesting that cerebrovascular senile patients will have Alzheimer's disease more often than patients without this condition.

There are no plausible clinical claims or reports that patients with Alzheimer's disease ever recover spontaneously. For this reason double-blind studies would be a waste of time and money, since it is illogical to use this method when a condition has no natural recovery rate. Instead, each clinical report of a recovery must be taken very seriously.

During October 2007 Mary, age seventy-three, complained that under stress her memory failed, which made her depressed. She tended to become confused in space but she was still able to drive her car. Until her memory began to fail she had been able to deal with stress with little difficulty. She was advised to improve her intake of vitamins including niacin (1 gram after each of three meals) and minerals and to eliminate dairy products. One month later she was very much better. After ten months she wrote to express her gratitude for her recovery and said, "Since I started the healing process with vitamins, I have been able to survive in my home when my family had been trying to convince me to sell and move into an apartment. I've lived here thirty-two years and I love my garden and was able to walk four blocks to market. Twice each week I watch my flowers come up, and weed my garden. My family refers to Alzheimer's, yet I know I am more aware and confident than I have been for years. If I hadn't had my meeting with you I'd be in hospital and my house sold. With deep gratitude."

The universal rule that all crows are black is no longer a universal rule if one sees a crow that is white. The clinical belief that there can be no recovery from Alzheimer's is equally false.

Orthomolecular treatment tries to optimize shelter. In this case it was important for this woman to remain in her home, which had been her shelter for thirty-two years. I suspect she was more grateful for that than for any other single factor. The program also removed a negative factor: the dairy foods to which she had been reacting for many years. And, it allowed her to retain her dignity and made it easier to demand and to be treated with respect and decency by those around her. She did not respond to just one factor. Niacin was only one of the important factors, as a member of a therapeutic team of nutrients.

Identical twins are ideal for comparison controlled trials. In animal studies it is recognized that one identical twin pair is equivalent to two groups containing forty nonrelated animals. Therefore, what happened to an identical-twin pair of women is very instructive. In this case, one twin developed galloping Alzheimer's and died within a few years. Her identical twin sister then started on a comprehensive megavitamin program. She lived another thirty years, mentally normal, and then died of a stroke.

If Alzheimer's patients have too little dopamine and therefore too little dopachrome, it would make sense to treat them by giving them safe amounts of L-dopa and yet protecting them against excessive dopachrome formation. This would include using L-dopa as if they were Parkinson's cases combined with at least three grams of niacin daily as the two main nutrients, with adequate amounts of calcium and magnesium and the elimination of aluminum. Of course the entire orthomolecular program would be even better.

Alzheimer's, Schizophrenia, and Down Syndrome

From my experience treating over 5,000 schizophrenic patients since 1952, I can not remember having seen any schizophrenic patients develop Alzheimer's disease. (Of course, it is possible that Alzheimer's disease may be found in the chronic populations in mental hospitals, with whom I have not had nearly as much experience.) Nor would I have expected it, as schizophrenia had been identified as a disease with no known metabolic dysfunction, and Alzheimer's disease was known to be caused by brain damage; an organic rather than a functional disorder. In 1952 one of the

Henry Turkel, M.D. (1903–1992)
Orthomolecular Medicine Hall of Fame 2007

I know Dr. Turkel, and I can testify to his sincerity and conviction. The results that he reports are striking. There is evidence that the patients would receive significant benefit.
—LINUS PAULING, PH.D.

It was thirty-five years ago that Dr. Henry Turkel testified before the United States Senate Select Committee on Nutrition and Human Needs. His presentation was entitled, "Medical Amelioration of Down's Syndrome Incorporating the Orthomolecular Approach." Dr. Turkel was the very voice of experience, having pioneered the nutritional treatment for Down's syndrome in the 1940s. Since then, he had successfully employed a combination of vitamins and other nutrients, plus some medication, with over 5,000 patients. In addition, Dr. Turkel wrote two key books: *Medical Treatment of Down Syndrome and Genetic Diseases* and *New Hope for the Mentally Retarded*.

Abram Hoffer has written:

"I first became interested in Down syndrome when I heard about the work being done by Dr. Henry Turkel in Detroit many years ago. I published many of his papers in the *Journal of Orthomolecular Psychiatry* and its earlier versions. Dr. Turkel suffered the fate of almost all early pioneers. He had the nerve to make his claims when everyone 'knew' that children with genetic defects could not possibly be treated successfully."

Linus Pauling specifically recognized Dr. Turkel's work in his book, *How to Live Longer and Feel Better:*

"The physician who has made the greatest effort to ameliorate Down syndrome is Dr. Henry Turkel of Detroit, Michigan . . . I know Dr. Turkel, and I can testify to his sincerity and conviction. The results that he reports are striking. Many of the children show a reduction of developmental abnormalities, especially of the bones. Their appearance changes in the direction of normalcy. Their mental ability and behavior improve to such an extent that they are able to hold jobs and support themselves. Rapid growth (increase in height) occurs during the period when tablets are being taken, and the growth stops during the periods when they are not taken. My conclusion is that there is little danger that this treatment or treatment with supplementary nutrients would do harm, and there is evidence that the patients would receive significant benefit. . . . I think that all (people with Down syndrome)—especially the younger ones—should try nutritional supplementation to see to what extent it benefits them."[26]

Used with permission of the Linus Pauling Institute, Oregon State University.

Jack Challem writes: "Vitamin therapy in Down syndrome began in 1940, when Henry Turkel, M.D., of Detroit became interested in treating the metabolic disorders of Down syndrome with a mixture of vitamins, minerals, fatty acids, digestive enzymes, lipotropic nutrients, glutamic acid, thyroid hormone, antihistamines, nasal decongestants, and a diuretic. By the 1950s he had devoted his practice almost entirely to Down syndrome patients, of whom he kept exceptionally detailed records, including serial photographs of their progress. Conventional medicine ignored Dr. Turkel and he eventually retired and moved to Israel. Turkel clearly demonstrated that one of the 'worst' genetic defects—trisomy, leading to Down syndrome—could be modified through what is largely a nutritional program with moderately high-dose supplements. The program never corrected the basic genetic defects in Down syndrome, of course, but it did correct much of the collateral biochemical consequences, leading to improvements in cognition, physical health, and appearance. Turkel was probably the first to show that nutrition could improve genetic programming, and that genetic predeterminism was limited."

For further reading:

Turkel, H. "Medical amelioration of Down syndrome incorporating the orthomolecular approach." *J Orthomolecular Psych* 4 (1975):102–115.

Turkel, H. "Medical amelioration of Down syndrome incorporating the orthomolecular approach," in: *Diet Related to Killer Diseases* V. *Nutrition and Mental Health.* Hearing before the Select Committee on Nutrition and Human Needs of the United States Senate, Washington, DC: U.S. Government Printing Office, 1977: 291–304.

Turkel, H. *Medical treatment of Down syndrome and genetic diseases,* Southfield, MI: Ubiotica, 4th rev. ed., 1985.

Turkel, H. *New hope for the mentally retarded: Stymied by the FDA.* New York, NY: Vantage Press, 1972.

patients in our psychiatric ward had been diagnosed with Alzheimer's disease. After a few weeks of observation he was sent to the closest mental hospital for permanent care, but a few weeks after he arrived his behavior became decidedly uncharacteristic of Alzheimer's disease. He became very aggressive and difficult, and he was rediagnosed as schizophrenic. He was given niacin, which we had just obtained, and he recovered. He surely had not had Alzheimer's disease.

Schizophrenia is characterized by major changes in perception and in thinking, with little memory loss, disorientation, and confusion. Organic psychosis is characterized by severe loss of memory, by disorientation with respect to time, place, and identity, and by confusion. Alzheimer's may also be confused with depression in the elderly. In my first-year residency in psychiatry in 1951, one of my patients clearly suffered from senile psychosis. I did not know how he might be treated. Dr. KcKerracher suggested I give him electroconvulsive therapy (ECT). This made no sense to me, but I went along with this advice. The patient made a complete recovery after having been demented for two years. I was really astonished at his recovery. Given the difficulty in diagnosing Alzheimer's disease, the failure to see any of the elderly chronic schizophrenic patients in my practice develop Alzheimer's is striking.

Down syndrome is a congenital condition that is associated with Alzheimer's disease. Alzheimer's tends to come early in these patients. Down patients also tend to suffer from depression more often, but the coexistence with schizophrenia is low. Three studies showed the following relationship: in the first study, 6 out of 371 Down patients had schizophrenia, and in the next two studies, of 119 and 315 patients, none were schizophrenic. From a total of 805 patients with Down syndrome, only 6 were also suffering from schizophrenia. Diagnosing schizophrenia in Down patients may be very difficult and the precise relationship between the two conditions may not be known, but it is clear that Down syndrome and Alzheimer's disease resemble each other a lot more than either resembles schizophrenia.

Dr. H. Turkel began to treat Down children early in the 1950s with a multivitamin, multimineral mixture plus thyroid. The results he saw and published, including pictures of recovered young patients, were very impressive. Dr Turkel believed that properly treated Down syndrome children would not suffer from early Alzheimer's. His work was not taken seriously and the Food and Drug Administration (FDA) made very strenuous attempts to suppress this treatment. Eventually he was able to use his preparation legally only in Michigan, as long as the product did not cross state lines. Dr. Turkel was embittered by this blatant attempt to keep these children sick. Sporadic half-hearted attempts were made to confirm his evidence with mixed results. Dr. B. Rimland concluded, after examining the literature, that Dr. Turkel's method was not fairly followed by other researchers who denied his conclusions. Dr Turkel is in the Orthomolecular Hall of Fame.

Thiel concluded, "Whether or not specifically due to the presence of a third 21st chromosome, metabolic disturbances are involved with Down syndrome. The nutritional profiles of the Down syndrome population do, in certain significant ways, differ from those of the general public. Various signs and symptoms associated with Down syndrome have been reported to improve when certain nutritional protocols have been tried (and there is no accepted medical treatment currently in existence for Down syndrome). Orthomolecular medicine has safely been treating people with Down syndrome for over sixty years. Orthomolecular medicine is a logical therapy to consider when Down syndrome is present."[25]

MacLeod is in full agreement with this conclusion. In his excellent 2003 book, *Down Syndrome and Vitamin Therapy*,[27] he recorded the phenomenal improvement seen in Down children when they were treated with the correct nutrients. He has advanced since Turkel in that his laboratory has been using some of the latest clinical laboratory tests to determine which of the nutrients have to be emphasized. The stories of some of the young people and their pictures offer proof that the orthomolecular approach pioneered by Dr. Turkel so many years ago is valid. As in so many other areas the medical establishment has once again shown a remarkable tendency to back the wrong horse.

Recently the findings by Li and his colleagues raised this question: Do schizophrenic patients get Alzheimer's disease? These researchers suggested that "Our findings have important implications for understanding protein deposition diseases, support the hypothesis that a common molecular mechanism may underlie development of pathological features of Parkinson's disease and Alzheimer's disease and suggests that common strategies of intervention could benefit patients suffering from these diseases"[28]. The adrenochrome hypothesis suggests that if schizophrenic patients have too much adrenochrome or dopachrome (from dopamine) this would protect them from the excessive formation of amyloid.

Religa and his coworkers reported levels of amyloid ß-peptide in the postmortem brains of schizophrenic and normal patients with and without Alzheimer's disease. They concluded that "In contrast to elderly schizophrenia patients with Alzheimer's disease pathology, those without Alzheimer's disease had amyloid ß-peptide levels that were not significantly different from those of normal subjects; hence amyloid ß-peptide does not account for the cognitive deficits in this group. These results suggest that the causes of cognitive impairment in 'pure' schizophrenia are different from those in Alzheimer's disease."[29] Seven of the brains came from patients with the dual diagnosis.

In a 1998 study, Purohit and colleagues examined 100 consecutive autopsy brain specimens of patients aged 52 to 101 years (mean age 76.5 years), 47 patients with nonschizophrenic psychiatric disorders from the same psychiatric hospital, and 50 age-matched control subjects. "Although 72% of the patients with schizophrenia showed cognitive impairment, AD [Alzheimer's disease] was diagnosed in only 9% of the patients and other dementing diseases were diagnosed in only 4% of the patients. The degree of senile plaques or neurofibrillary tangles was not different in the group with schizophrenia compared with the age-matched controls or the group with nonschizophrenic psychiatric disorders" They concluded, "This study provides evidence that elderly patients with schizophrenia are not inordinately prone to the development of AD or to increased senile plaques or neurofibrillary tangle formation in the brain. Other dementing neurodegenerative disorders are also uncommon. The cognitive impairment in elderly patients with schizophrenia must, therefore, be related to some alternative mechanisms."[30]

Anxiety

In my (AH) very first book on niacin in 1962, I discussed what little was then known of vitamin B$_3$ as a sedative in Chapter 3. The old term "sedative," which applied to the barbiturates, has been replaced by the term "antianxiety." The first report of niacin's antianxiety properties appeared in 1949, when it was reported that it was synergistic with some drugs. Later I found that it indeed had anticonvulsive properties if combined with anticonvulsants, and it was possible to achieve better control with less sedation by adding niacin to the anticonvulsant program. I also found that niacin increased the sedative effect of phenobarbital, a very common barbiturate, when they were combined. Further studies showed that it was also therapeutic for a mix of anxiety and depression and agitation. I have seen this frequently over the past fifty years. Niacin also sedated animals when a sufficient amount was administered.

Prousky described the orthomolecular treatment of anxiety in 2006.[31] Vitamin B$_3$ is a major factor in this program. Currently the press and perhaps the public as well have recognized that the xenobiotic antidepressants used to treat depression and anxiety are seldom better than placebo. In addition, they are very addictive and toxic because the withdrawal effects are so severe and prolonged. Physicians concerned about the use of these drugs should study Prousky's book. They will be reassured that orthomolecular treatment of anxiety and depression is much more effective without the use of these dangerous drugs. Over the past ten years I have not started anyone on these drugs—indeed, I have done just the opposite. Most of these patients came because they wanted to eliminate them from their program.

Cancer

Niacin is effective in decreasing the death rate of patients with cancer by protecting cells and tissues from damage by toxic molecules or free radicals. One of the most exciting findings is that *niacin will help protect against cancer.* A 1987 conference at Texas College of Osteopathic Medicine in Fort Worth was already the eighth conference to discuss niacin and cancer. The first was held in Switzerland in 1984.

In the body, niacin is converted to nicotinamide adenine dinucleotide (NAD). NAD is a coenzyme necessary to many reactions. Another enzyme, poly (Adenosine adenine phosphate ribose) polymerase, uses NAD to catalyze the formation of ADP-ribose. The poly (ADP-ribose) polymerase is activated by strands of DNA that have been broken by smoke, herbicides, and other toxins. When the long chains of DNA are damaged, poly (ADP-ribose) helps repair it by unwinding the damaged protein. Poly (ADP-ribose) also increases the activity of DNA ligase. This enzyme cuts off the damaged strands of DNA and increases the ability of the cell to repair itself after exposure to carcinogens.

Jacobson and Jacobson[32,33] discussed the anti-cancer properties of niacin at the Texas conference. They believe niacin (more specifically, NAD) prevents processes that lead to cancer. They found that *one group of human cells given enough niacin and then exposed to carcinogens developed cancer at a rate only one-tenth of the rate in the same cells not given niacin.*

It is not surprising that niacin also decreased the death rate from cancer in the National Coronary Drug Study. I gave both niacin, 3 grams per day, and ascorbic acid, 3 grams per day, to the first cancer patient I treated in 1960. He was psychotic and had been admitted to our psychiatric ward, Royal University Hospital in Saskatoon, Saskatchewan. I did not realize that I would see him recover from both of his diseases, the psychosis and his inoperable lung cancer.[34]

Cancer, the Mauve Factor, and Niacin

We (AH and colleagues) discovered a substance in the urine of psychiatric patients that we called the mauve factor, as it stained the paper chromatograms mauve.[35] For comparison we analyzed the urine of normal subjects and patients suffering very severe stress, such as terminal cancer. A psychotic delirious seventy-five-year-old man with terminal lung cancer was admitted to the psychiatric ward. He had been treated with cobalt bomb radiation, and the cancer clinic concluded that he could not live more than a month or two. He excreted huge quantities of the mauve factor. Most of the lung cancer patients I tested excreted this substance in large amounts.

By then I knew from our previous therapeutic trials that psychiatric patients who excreted the mauve factor responded very well to treatment with large doses of vitamin B_3, (niacin or niacinamide). I suggested to his resident that he start him on niacin, 3 grams daily. The patient was started on niacin on a Friday, and by the following Monday he was mentally normal. I was interested in seeing what the long-term effect of the vitamin would be on his psychiatric state. I offered to give him both niacin and vitamin C for free if he would come to my office each month to obtain it.

A year later I was surprised when I was told by the cancer clinic that they could no longer see any lesions in his lung. Every three months they had seen a reduction in the size of his cancer. He died twenty-eight months after I started him on the vitamin. No autopsy was performed. I thought the niacin might have been the most important agent in the reduction of his cancer, since it was and still is my favorite vitamin. I had added vitamin C only because I did so routinely for my schizophrenic patients. The exciting work of Cameron and Pauling, however, suggested that the vitamin C was the more important single factor, but since then I included niacin in my program for treating cancers.[36]

Niacin and Chemotherapy

Recent studies have increased my confidence that niacin is important for cancer treatment. In 2008 Bartleman, Jacobs, and Kirkland[37] found that niacin supplementation in rats helped protect them from the long-term deleterious effect of chemotherapy, especially the nonlymphocitic leukemia. Secondary or treatment-related cancer occurs in 5 to 15 percent of chemotherapy patients due to DNA damage. Jacobson[38] reported studies of DNA damage in cultured mouse and human cells low in niacin, suggesting that niacin may be protective against cancer. She used a biochemical method based on the observation that with deficient niacin, NAD readily decreases and NADP remains relatively constant. She used the following algorithm to determine a "niacin number," which would indicate a healthy versus low level of niacin in the body: (NAD/NAD + NADP) x 100% from whole. Healthy controls showed a mean niacin number of 62.8 +/- 3.0. Analyses of women in the Malmo Diet and Cancer Study showed a mean niacin number of 60.4 with a range of 44 to 75, with an unpredictably large number of individuals having low values.

Moalem[39] reported that methylation (addition of a CH3 group) of genes is related to cancer. Investigators found a very high correlation between breast cancer recurrence and the amount of methylation of a gene called PITX2. In breast cancer patients with low methylation rates, 90 percent were free of cancer for ten years, while patients with high methylation rates only 65 percent remained cancer free for that length of time. (Smoking increases methylation as does chewing betel nut, since both are carcinogenic.) Niacin provides one of a few natural powerful methyl acceptors in the body. Jacobs and Kirkland's very important observations strongly suggest that every patient receiving chemotherapy should also be given niacin. Oncologists are not overly accustomed to seeing recoveries. If they want to improve the outcome of treatment, they should not continue to ignore this work.[40–43]

Schizophrenia, Niacin, and Cancer

Dr. Foster and I (AH) discussed a hypothesis regarding why schizophrenic patients do not get cancer as frequently as patients who are not schizophrenic We suggest that excess production of adrenochrome, a derivative of adrenalin, creates the psychosis, as it is a hallucinogen. At the same time, it also protects them against cancer, as it is an inhibitor of cell mitosis. Out of about five thousand patients I have seen since 1955, only twelve developed cancer. One developed cancer only recently, fifty years after being cured from her schizophrenia. The literature does not show such a clear differentiation. My patients were all on niacin and most were also on vitamin C, while none of the literature series were. This might explain this difference. In other words, these vitamins protected these patients from cancer. Of the two vitamins, niacin is probably the more relevant because the amount of vitamin C given was three grams daily or less. But when my patients were treated with large doses of vitamin C, all but one recovered.

Skin Cancer, Sunscreen, and Niacinamide

Now here's something you may not have been expecting: recently Professor Darmian and colleagues reported that niacinamide was a better sunscreen against ultraviolet-induced cancers than the common sunscreens.[44] It protects against both UVA and UVB, while common sunscreens do not protect against UVA. Niacinamide does so by maintaining the immune defenses of the skin against ultraviolet radiation. If this vitamin can protect against melanoma, it becomes even more probable that it will protect against other cancers. Of course the entire orthomolecular program, including selenium and antioxidants such as vitamin E and C, will provide even more protection. The common sunscreens decrease exposure to ultraviolet and therefore reduce the production of vitamin D_3 in the skin. This increases the number of people who will suffer from lack of vitamin D, especially because we are exposed to so many warnings about the dangers of the sun and the need to lather ourselves with these preparations. Niacinamide does not prevent the body from making vitamin D.

Cancer of the Stomach

In September 2008, a woman consulted with me (AH) to get nutritional advice for her stomach cancer. She had been treated for colon cancer six years earlier with the usual three components of modern cancer therapy (chemotherapy, radiation, and surgery) and was apparently well for five years. Then cancer of her stomach was diagnosed. She had surgery but no further treatment was offered. As I listened to her story I could not help but wonder whether she would have had this second cancer if she had been given niacin when she was originally treated for her colon cancer. It could not have hurt her and may have saved her from terminal cancer.

Late-Effect Cancer and Niacin

The Canadian Cancer Society reports that two-thirds of children who survive after cancer treatment have one or more late-effect cancers, and of these, one-third are grave or life-threatening, including damage to the heart, lungs, and stomach.[45] The risk of later cancers is mentioned, but not the secondary cancers induced by radiation or chemotherapy. These may average around 10 percent of the total. This article discusses what is being done to decrease these late-effect cancers, but the use of niacin in conjunction with the original treatment is not mentioned.

To understand why niacin can help to reduce cancer risk, it is necessary to understand a little biochemistry. Niacin, niacinamide and nicotinamide adenine dinucleotide (NAD) are interconvertible via a pyridine nucleotide cycle. NAD, the coenzyme, is hydrolyzed or split into niacinamide and adenosine dinucleotide phosphate (ADP-ribose). Niacinamide is converted into niacin, which in turn is once more built into NAD. The enzyme which splits ADP is known as poly (ADP-ribose) polymerase, or poly (ADP) synthetase, or poly (ADP-ribose) transferase.

Poly (ADP-ribose) polymerase is activated when strands of deoxyribonucleic acid (DNA) are broken. The enzyme transfers NAD to the ADP-ribose polymer, binding it onto a number of proteins. The poly (ADP-ribose) activated by DNA breaks helps repair such breaks by unwinding the nucleosomal structure of damaged chromatids. It also may increase the activity of DNA ligase. This enzyme cuts damaged ends off strands of DNA and increases the cell's capacity to repair itself. Damage caused by any carcinogenic factor such as radiation or chemicals is, as a result, neutralized or counteracted. Jacobson and Jacobson hypothesized that this is why niacin can protect against cancer. They illustrated this by treating two groups of human cells with carcinogens. The group given adequate niacin developed tumors at a rate of only 10 percent of that seen in the group that was deficient in niacin. Dr. M. Jacobson is quoted as saying, "We know that diet is a major risk factor, that diet has both beneficial and detrimental components. What we cannot assess at this point is the optimal amount of niacin in the diet. . . . The fact that we don't have pellagra does not mean we are getting enough niacin to confer resistance to cancer."[46] About 20 mg per day of niacin will prevent pellagra in people who are not chronic pellagrins. The latter may require twenty-five times as much niacin to remain free of pellagra.

For more information about niacin and cancer, see the report from the Linus Pauling Institute available at http://lpi.oregonstate.edu/infocenter/vitamins/niacin.

Cataracts

Larger than dietary quantities of all of the B-complex vitamins, including niacin, appear to help prevent cataracts, as does vitamin A. A study of 2,873 persons taking supplemental amounts of these nutrients showed a 30 to 60 percent reduction in nuclear or cortical cataracts.[47]

Antioxidants such as lutein and vitamins C and E are also important for cataract prevention. A review of the literature recommended that people take "considerably higher than the current recommended daily intakes"[48] of vitamin C and four times the RDA of vitamin E.

Cholera and Diarrhea

Niacin is protective in a strikingly large variety of diseases. Niacin also inhibits and reverses intestinal secretion caused by the cholera toxin and E. coli enterotoxin. A randomized controlled clinical trial showed that 2,000 mg of niacin per day, in divided doses, reduced fluid loss in cholera patients. It did so in less than half a day, and was described as "well-tolerated" by patients.[49] Niacin also reduces diarrhea associated with pancreatic tumors in man. Niacinamide does not appear to have this fluid-loss reducing effect.[50]

Detoxification

L. Ron Hubbard, the controversial founder of Scientology, combined induced sweating by heat (for example, sauna) with niacin as a way of treating patients. Each technique by itself has been widely used with no danger and with many positive effects. It is clear that niacin is safe and effective. Sweating lodges have been and are being used by native North Americans as part of a well established ritual. It has been found to be very effective. Hubbard put these two treatments together by placing patients on niacin and then having them use heat to induce sweating. The method has been helpful, but the Hubbard detoxification program has been vilified and critically condemned simply because Hubbard was the original proponent. The main criticism is that his explanations for why it works are not scientific. I (AH) find this criticism rather simplistic, since the entire psychiatric profession has accepted psychoanalysis for many years although it has not been shown to work and has some very bizarre explanations to explain why it should work. Logically, the only important questions for any program of therapy are, "Does it work?" and, "Is it safe?" If it is eventually shown to be effective it will be easy to develop hypotheses, most of which will be wrong, to explain why. We have never been short of explanations like the stress hypothesis of peptic ulcers, which in the vast majority of cases turned out to be caused by an infection. The battle over Hubbard's detoxification treatment is a matter of one church called Medicine attacking another church called Scientology. You might wonder what happened to evidence-based medicine, until you realize that to be accepted as evidence the work has to come from a prestigious institution like Harvard, has to be done by well-established scientists, has to be published in standard journals (whose club of editorial committees keep out really new ideas), has to be accepted by the governing bodies of the traditional medical profession, and, of course, must be double-blind.

Epidermolysis Bullosa

In *Harrison's Principles of Internal Medicine*,[51] an inherited zinc deficiency disease is described. The symptoms and signs include severe chronic diarrhea, muscle wasting, alopecia (loss of hair), and rough, thick, ulcerated skin around the body orifices and on the extremities.

CC came to see me on December 19, 1989 and was seen for the second and last time January 5, 1990. A few days after he was born in June 1972, his skin, which had been under pressure from a forceps delivery, began to slough off. A few days later lesions, which later blistered, developed on his face, mouth, chest, and limbs. He was treated with topical antibiotics using sterile techniques but did not improve. The lesions in his mouth made it impossible for him to feed, and he became anemic and hypoproteinemic. One month later he was diagnosed with epidermolysis bullosa and started on vitamin E, 600 IU orally, later increased to 800 IU. At age four months, 200 mg of ascorbic acid was added, and at age six months he was given iron supplementation and the vitamin E was increased to 1,000 IU. There was no response. He was then admitted to the hospital suffering from stomatitis, and again, in April 1973, for gastroenteritis and pneumonia. By now he had multiple lesions, denuded areas on his legs, no nails, adhesions between his fingers and toes. On top of this he was constantly constipated. His mother had to remove his stools manually daily, and in 1986 he was admitted to the hospital to have his stools removed. In 1980 his parents took him to West Germany for two and one-half months to be treated by a biochemist, who was using special skin salves and other treatment with some success. He was placed on a vegetarian diet supplemented with a moderate vitamin program (doses unknown). This regimen was helpful. They went back to Germany once more for ten days and would have gone again, but they could no longer afford to do so.

When I first saw CC he appeared to be about ten years old, very short and immature. Mentally he appeared to be normal. There were no perceptual changes or thought disorder, and his mood was surprisingly cheerful and upbeat. The bullous lesions continued to erupt. He had lost all of his fingers and toes. An attempt had been made to separate them surgically in Italy with no success. He did tell me that food did not taste normal. He was still severely constipated. To test his sense of taste for a possible zinc deficiency, I gave him a teaspoon of a special zinc sulfate solution. He found it tasted like stale water, not bitter as it would to normal individuals. I could not order a blood test for zinc since all his superficial veins were gone and it would have required a cut down. Zinc deficiency will cause dwarfism, retarded wound healing, and loss of taste. The classic response to chronic zinc deficiency is acrodermatitis enteropathica (AE). AE babies develop infections around their body orifices.

I advised that CC start on the following supplements: niacinamide, 500 mg twice daily; ascorbic acid, 500 mg three times daily (1,500 mg, about 100 times the RDA); pyridoxine, 100 mg twice daily; cod liver oil, one-half teaspoon daily; ten drops twice daily of a solution of zinc sulfate 10% with manganese chloride 1/2%; plus 1 teaspoon of linseed oil daily to increase his intake of omega-3 essential fatty acids.

Two weeks later he was much improved. His mood remained normal but his parents were much more cheerful. In that brief period he had grown half an inch in height, his skin was much healthier, and the lesions appeared about one-third as frequently. Those that did develop healed much more quickly. He had gained two pounds. He was no longer constipated and was able to have normal bowel movements for the first time in his life.

This patient's rapid response does not prove it was due entirely to the administration of the zinc. I suspect that zinc was the main therapeutic variable, but the other nutrients must also have played an important part.

I spoke to his pediatrician on October 17, 1991. She had just seen him a week before. She told me that his skin condition was stable, but that he had started to show emotional problems as he matured. CC called me on October 24, 1991. He said that his skin condition was stable even though he had remained on the total nutrient approach for only one year. Since then he had minor skin eruptions in the spring and in the fall. He had grown about three to four inches and had gained fifteen pounds. He was still constipated. His mood was level and he was cheerful. He died November 1998 from a bowel obstruction.

Fatigue

Diagnosing fatigue is very difficult, as being tired accompanies almost every known affliction from which so many of us suffer. Fatigue is a universal response to being sick, and is advantageous from an evolutionary point of view. It is a warning and forces us to decrease our activity so the body can devote more energy to healing itself. Fatigue is common in all nutritional diseases including starvation, deficiency, and dependencies; with all infections; with lack of rest and sleep; with diseases such as diabetes, multiple sclerosis (MS), and muscle disease; with chronic pain; with diagnosable cancer; and even in manic patients who do not appear to be tired but will admit they are. Fatigue is common to mood disorders and schizophrenia, and of course is made much worse by the modern antipsychotic drugs. I think the term fatigue should be reserved only for patients with no identified causes for their symptoms and suggest they be diagnosed with idiopathic fatigue (IF).

There is a cause for chronic fatigue in every sufferer that has to be identified. One of the major causes of idiopathic fatigue has been ignored. This is the hypothesis developed by the New Zealand biologist Les Simpson. Maupin's brief review of Simpson's research is excellent.[52] Simpson showed that impaired blood flow was a major factor in many chronic diseases which create chronic fatigue. Decreased blood viscosity and decreased capillary blood flow are involved. Since becoming aware of his work, I have found that his therapeutic program using essential fatty acids and large doses of vitamin B_{12}, to which I have added niacin, very effective in treating many cases of IF. If the diameters of the capillaries are too small, they cannot deliver enough blood to the tissues. Associated reasons are the size and shape of the red blood cells, which slows down their movement through the capillaries. Red blood cells do not flow through these small vessels; they crawl or wiggle through. This makes sense, as this process facilitates the transfer of gases from the inner lining of the capillaries to the red blood cells. In abnormal conditions the cells may be too large, as in pernicious anemia, or they may be misshapen, and they may be too rigid. They must be flexible in order to transverse the capillaries. Simpson demonstrated these changes in many studies in chronic diseases such as MS.

Niacin and Fatigue

Ed Boyle, one of the first physicians to take our niacin findings seriously, discovered that some of the capillaries in the retina were empty in some patients. He became interested in the sludging (clumping) of red blood cells, which made it difficult for them to traverse the capillaries. Red blood cells have to go through the capillaries individually, not holding hands with their neighbors. He thought that these cells had lost some of their surface electronegative charge and were no longer able to repel each other. Based on Boyle's theory I developed my program for IF, which follows:

- Large doses of parenteral vitamin B_{12} (1 to 5 milligrams of hydroxocobalamin), up to several times each week, and gradually decreasing the frequency as the patient improved. This vitamin would decrease the size of the red cells.

- Essential fatty acids to increase the flexibility of the red cell surface membrane. Boyle used evening primrose oil; I use the fish oils, which are richer in omega-3 essential fatty acids.

- Niacin—up to 1 gram three times daily (that is, up to 3,000 mg total), after each of three meals. This breaks up the clumps of red cells by keeping them from sticking to each other. It also dilates the capillaries (via the flush or vasodilatation) and allows more blood to traverse them. There is an additional advantage. Simpson points out that when plasma cholesterol levels are raised, there is an increase in the cholesterol content of the red cell membrane. This change results in the red cells becoming less pliable, which reduces capillary blood flow.[53,54] Increased cholesterol levels are associated with increased blood viscosity.

This program increases the flow of blood to the tissues of the body by dilating the capillaries; deceasing the size of the larger red blood cells, making them more flexible; breaking up and preventing sludging of the cells; and decreasing viscosity. The results have been spectacular. It is possible to spot a person whose blood is sludged by their appearance. They are obese, very pale, sweaty, and short of breath. Often after the first dose of niacin their normal color returns. Patients find this program easy to follow. Perhaps this type of IF should be called blood rheology fatigue.

The above program is the specific treatment for rheology fatigue, but it is not the ideal treatment for IF. The best treatment for IF is the program that works so well for the pandeficiency syndrome (see Chapter 6). The ideal program includes finding and dealing with the cause or causes of the fatigue. Nutritionally, it includes good nutrition free of the sugars, sweeteners, and foods that one is allergic to. It also includes vitamin C, selenium, essential fatty acids, vitamin D (especially in northern countries), calcium and magnesium, and quite often zinc. A female patient of mine with chronic fatigue and fibromyalgia along with depression, anxiety, and fear started on this program. By the end of the second year she was normal and delighted with how well she was feeling. She had been started on vitamin D, 6,000 IU daily, but only after she increased the dose to 10,000 IU did her fibromyalgia suddenly clear. After a while she went back to 6,000 IU. The pain did not return.

Hartnup Disease

Hartnup disease is due to a hereditary inability to absorb tryptophan and some other amino acids. It is an uncommon condition that results in a skin rash and some brain abnormalities. Either niacin or niacinamide will provide relief from skin and neurological symptoms of this fairly rare, inherited disorder. Supplementation is essential, as dietary quantities of niacin are insufficient and ineffective.[55] Dosage recommendations vary; somewhere in the vicinity of 300 mg or more per day is probably optimum.

Huntington's Disease

Huntington's disease is a mixture of schizophrenic symptoms and neurological signs and symptoms. It is quite rare. I (AH) have seen two cases, and they both recovered on a combination of niacin, which protects them from the psychosis, and vitamin E, which protects them against the physical symptoms. This is a series of only two patients, with a 100 percent success rate. Dr. Tenna wrote to me that she had three patients doing quite well. "The niacin is the key to energy, it seems. Even the sibling who is most affected is responding to activated B$_3$, B vitamins, coenzyme Q$_{10}$ (CoQ$_{10}$), and folate (5mg tds[three times daily])."

Migraine Headache

There has been interest in using niacin to treat and prevent migraine headaches since 1951.[56] Recently, the Mayo Clinic Division of Pain Management in Scottsdale, Arizona described "a patient whose migraine headaches responded dramatically to sustained-release niacin as preventive treatment. Niacin is not generally considered to be effective for migraine prevention. However, low plasma levels of serotonin have been implicated in migraine pathogenesis, and niacin may act as a negative feedback regulator on the kynurenine pathway to shunt tryptophan into the serotonin pathway, thus increasing plasma serotonin levels. Sustained-release niacin merits further study as a potentially useful preventive therapy for migraine headache."[57]

A 2005 review of nine articles investigating niacin therapy for migraine stated: "Intravenous and oral niacin has been employed in the treatment of acute and chronic migraine and tension-type headaches, but its use has not become part of contemporary medicine, nor have there been randomized controlled trials further assessing this novel treatment. . . . Hypothetical reasons for niacin's effectiveness include its vasodilatory properties, and its ability to improve mitochondrial energy metabolism. . . . Although niacin's mechanisms of action have not been substantiated from controlled clinical trials, this agent may have beneficial effects upon migraine and tension-type headaches."[58]

Multiple Sclerosis

New research confirms that niacinamide, also known as vitamin B$_3$, is a key to the successful treatment of multiple sclerosis (MS) and other nerve diseases. Niacinamide, say researchers at Harvard Medical School, "profoundly prevents the degeneration of demyelinated axons and improves the behavioral deficits."[59] Kaneko and coworkers found that nicotinamide, by increasing NAD levels in the nervous system, was therapeutic against MS in the mouse model. It prevented further degeneration of axons and inflammation of the axons and loss of myelin. A Reuters News report added that "Dr. Abram Hoffer, who was not involved in the research and is in practice in Saskatoon, Saskatchewan, has treated over sixty MS patients over the years with large oral doses of vitamin B$_3$ ranging from 3 to 6 grams per day. 'In most cases, when the treatment was started early, early results were very good,' he said."[60]

This is very good news, but it is not at all new news. Over sixty years ago, Canadian physician H.T. Mount began treating multiple sclerosis patients with intravenous B$_1$ (thiamine) plus intramuscular liver extract, which provides other B vitamins. He followed the progress of these patients for up to twenty-seven years. The results were excellent and were described in a paper published in the *Canadian Medical Association Journal* in 1973.[61]

Mount was not alone. Forty years ago, Frederick Robert Klenner, M.D., of North Carolina, was using vitamins B$_3$ and B$_1$, along with the rest of the B-complex vitamins, vitamins C and E, and other nutrients including magnesium, calcium, and zinc to arrest and reverse multiple sclerosis.[62,63] Klenner's complete treatment program was originally published as "Treating Multiple Sclerosis Nutritionally," in *Cancer Control Journal*.[64] His detailed megavitamin protocol is posted at http://www.tldp.com/issue/ 11_00/klenner.htm.

Dr. Mount and Dr. Klenner were persuaded by their clinical observations that multiple sclerosis, myasthenia gravis, and many other neurological disorders were primarily due to nerve cells being starved of nutrients. Each physician tested this theory by giving his patients large, orthomolecular quantities of nutrients. Their successful cures over decades of medical practice proved that their theory was correct. B-complex vitamins, including thiamine as well as niacinamide, are absolutely vital for nerve cell health. Where pathology already exists, unusually large quantities of vitamins are needed to repair damaged nerve cells.

Dr. Klenner used a combination of B-complex vitamins given by injection and orally to treat, and cure, many patients with MS. I (AH) have used a modification of the Klenner program, as many patients found it too difficult to obtain Dr. Klenner's preferred parenteral (intravenous) administration of vitamins. It is an effective treatment.

One man has gone public with his success story. Peter Leeds was diagnosed with multiple sclerosis in 2004. In October 2005, Dr. Hoffer put him on a high-protein but dairy-free diet, and had him take vitamin supplements including niacin, the rest of the B complex, vitamins C and D, zinc, and salmon oil. One year later, he was "very much better. The only thing left is some slight numbness in his fingers, but there is a major improvement. In fact he had several MRIs, and the second one showed a major deteriorating spot in his brain that is now almost gone, which was very surprising to the neurologist."[65]

And here is a November 2008 report from a client placed on treatment several years ago. He had the classical clinical and pathological changes in his brain and his prognosis was not good. "I just got the results of my latest MRI on Wednesday. It showed no progression of the disease since the previous MRIs of two years ago. The MS specialist was pretty pleased, and says I'm doing something right." He recovered after about one and a half years of treatment. The neurologist found him normal. The brain scan was normal. His doctor said that had he not seen the brain scan at first he would not have diagnosed him as having multiple sclerosis. Then, having pronounced him well, he asked the former patient whether he would participate in testing a new drug for treating MS! Pharmaceutical hope springs eternal.

Nephritis

Only one in ten patients who need kidney transplants gets one. There are too few kidneys available, and the operation is expensive: over $100,000 in the United States. Some 30,000 transplants are done in the United States each year; about 100,000 persons are on waiting lists. In 2005, 341,000 Americans were on dialysis. Dialysis costs approximately $50,000 per year. But there is potential solution. If diseased kidneys were cured, there would be no need for dialysis and transplants.

Kidney tissue is protected by niacinamide.[66] It protected rats against the diabetogenic effect of the antibiotic streptozotocin. Clinically, niacin has been used to successfully treat patients with severe glomerulonephritis, a condition that impairs normal kidney function and results in tissue swelling, high blood pressure, and blood in the urine. One of my (AH) patients was being readied for dialysis. Her nephrologist had advised her she would die if she refused to undergo this procedure. She started on niacin 3,000 mg per day and is still well, twenty-five years later.

Condorelli[67] listed a large number of cardiovascular problems he treated with niacin, including nephritis. About forty years ago a woman told me she had just been diagnosed with kidney failure. She would have to start dialysis immediately in preparation for a kidney transplant when one became available. Kidney dialysis had just been introduced to Saskatoon, and she was very worried. While she was telling me this I remembered the Italian studies, and suggested she discuss them with her doctor. I advised that it could do no harm and might help. She discussed the studies with her doctor, who thought the idea was hilarious. But it was no laughing matter for her. She rejected his advice and started on niacin on her own. Thirty years later, when we were having dinner in Victoria, her husband reminded me of this. She had recovered and remained well on niacin, three grams daily. Her recovery broke the rule that there was no treatment for nephritis.

Later Dr. Max Vogel, an orthomolecular physician in Calgary, told me about a similar case. A twelve-year-old girl with glomerulonephritis was given niacin by her father, a teacher. When no treatment was offered to her he researched as much as he could and discovered this vitamin. She recovered. He then had Dr. Vogel examine her. He confirmed that she had been sick and was now well. So now we have two cases out of two self-treated with niacin. As far as I know, no one else has tried this.

Two recoveries may not be very convincing to physicians raised on double-blind studies, but it is convincing to me and suggests that there must be other patients with nephritis who would also get well on this program. It is surely beyond all reason to conclude that these two recoveries, directly and indirectly known to me, would be the only cases on Earth. If one crow is white, it surely raises the odds that there are other crows that are white. In the same way, if one or two patients recover from a disease for which there is no treatment, it surely means there are other patients who will have the same results. But if no one looks into this, we will not know what proportion of the one-half million North Americans headed for kidney transplants can be helped. Think of the enormous savings to patients, families, and society if only one in a hundred were healed! But there is no incentive for Big Pharma to research this, as vitamin-based cures do not bring in billions of dollars in profit. The kidney transplant industry would be devastated if each patient has an average expenditure of only about $200 per year. Treating only ten patients successfully would save over a million dollars in treatment and maintenance costs—and given the 100 percent recovery experienced by our two patients, it is highly likely that the number of people who do get well would be much greater than ten.

Obesity

Many traditional nutritionists, who are strongly opposed to orthomolecular therapy and practice, promote the simple view that obesity is due to the very simple rule: too many calories in and too few calories expended out. This has become the standard belief of all anti-obesity programs because it seems to make so much sense. However, according to Taube, his massive examination of the clinical literature provides little support for this idea. There is no relation between the amount of food consumed and the amount of exercise expended and the absence or presence of obesity. Many people are not obese no matter how little or how much they eat, and too many are too fat no matter how little they eat. The problem is not the total amount but the kind of food consumed. According to Cleave, Yudkin, Taube, and many others, the main factor that creates obesity is the amount of sugar and refined carbohydrates that are eaten. Sugars and foods that rapidly release sugars into the blood are the villains.

It is true that if one eats too many calories there will a much greater tendency to put on weight, but the real question is: Why do these people eat too much junk food?

I (AH) think they do this because they are sick. An example is the intolerable weight gain of patients who are treated with Zyprexa, an atypical antipsychotic drug. I have seen young patients gain sixty pounds in six months after being placed on this dangerous psychiatric drug. It increases appetite enormously. But this is a relatively rare situation. A more common reason for obesity is the modern high-tech diet, which is deficient in every nutrient but contains plenty of sugars and a high proportion of refined foods. This combination creates an appetite to eat more. I call this theory the Wald hypothesis. George Wald got the Nobel Prize for his work with vitamin A. He also showed that starving rats were more active (ran a lot more) than rats on a normal diet, but rats on a diet with enough calories but none of the B vitamins also displayed increased running.[68] It makes sense that hunger will increase running (activity) in animals since that motivates them to seek food; to hunt. But it is surprising that depriving them of the B vitamins will do the same unless one postulates that the animals experience the B-vitamin deficiency as equivalent to hunger and try to deal with it by increasing activity. Dr. William Kaufman discussed how niacin deficiency causes decreased running in his 1949 book, *The Common Form of Joint Dysfunction.*[69] The diet too rich in sugars is also too deficient in B vitamins. Since during evolution animals who did not respond to hunger by searching for food would not be around today, activity became a natural genetic reflex. Thus the modern diet activates people in the same way.

There are three scenarios that relate insufficient nutrition to increased activity. The first is our modern high-tech diet, where no one starves, food is plentiful but deficient, and it is easily obtained. The hunger for nutrients (which the body identifies as food) increases appetite, leading to too much being eaten. As a result, people get fat, but they feel better because they are getting more of the B vitamins. People on a high-tech diet remain uncomfortable if they are forced to remain thin. In the second scenario there is not enough food. In this case, populations deficient in B vitamins will not be able to get the vitamins they need by eating more as there is no more to eat. These people will become lean and hyperactive until they are felled by starvation. In the third scenario, in children, the drive for the B vitamins increases activity and leads to the hyperactive syndrome and later to obesity.

The hypothesis that intake of calories from foods deficient in B vitamins increases activity, either by eating more and being more active, is easily tested. I have done so to a limited degree. I tried to help many obese patients with little success using any type of reducing diet. But they would lose weight with comfort when I advised them to go back to the stone-age diet, to take ample amounts of B vitamins, and to eat as little or as much as they wanted. This is not a reducing diet; it is a healthy lifestyle diet. That is the best approach to eliminating obesity.

Parkinsonism

Epidemiological evidence shows that Parkinson's disease is precipitated by trigger factors that activate the disease. The only effective, palliative treatment is L-dopa. It became the treatment of choice even though the original double-blind trials were not promising. The original researchers did not use a high enough dose, which supported the view that a deficiency of l-dopamine was responsible for Parkinson's disease. Later it was found that part of the brain was deficient in coenzyme Q_{10} and NAD. But unfortunately l-dopamine will be oxidized into l-dopachrome, which is toxic. It kills neurons and creates psychotic symptoms and signs. Foster and Hoffer discussed the psychotomimetic effects of L-dopa. They were also provided an explanation of Oliver Sacks' findings on the remarkable transient effect of L-dopa on patients with encephalitis lethargica, as dramatized in the film *Awakenings* (more on this below). Such huge doses of L-dopa are certainly very toxic to the brain.

On August 31, 2008, *Sixty Minutes* reported about improvement in patients who suffered from minimally conscious states (MCS). These patients retain some awareness even though they appear to have no consciousness. The program described one of the patients, who miraculously awakened after ten years and asked about his family. One of his doctors believes that he awakened after he was given an anti-Parkinsonism drug. This probably was L-dopa, but was not named on the program. A few others responded to a sleeping pill which normally puts people to sleep. If one hypothesizes that MCS patients are like the patients described by Oliver Sacks, this suggests that they should be treated with L-dopa and niacin. Since these compounds are not covered by patents and drug companies will therefore avoid them like the plague, it is time that investigators free themselves of their emotional and financial attachment to Big Pharma.

"Dr. Hoffer has discovered that high doses of niacin are very helpful in preventing Parkinson's psychosis. His use of this vitamin is based on the adrenochrome hypothesis of schizophrenia which has been described previously. Birkmayer et al. also found that both oral and parenteral NADH were equally effective in Parkinson's disease. They treated 885 patients with one or other of these methods and found that only about 20 percent did not benefit. Younger patients, who had not been symptomatic as long, responded better. To avoid damage in the stomach their oral preparation had to be stabilized. NADH in ordinary gelatin capsules was not effective, as had been found with NAD when treating schizophrenic patients."[70]

As Foster and Hoffer described in a 2004 *Medical Hypotheses* article, "The Two Faces of L-DOPA: Benefits and Adverse Side Effects in the Treatment of Encephalitis Lethargica, Parkinson's Disease, Multiple Sclerosis and

Amyotrophic Lateral Sclerosis,"[71] three measures must be addressed when treating Parkinson's disease. These are: dealing with oxidative stress (decreasing it where possible) and using natural antioxidants; giving natural methyl acceptors (the most readily available of which is vitamin B_3); and using high-dose antioxidants to mitigate the adverse toxic effects of L-dopa.

Sacks described treating twenty patients with L-dopa. The initial dose was 500 milligrams daily but, if required, was increased gradually to 6 grams. Many patients showed great early progress, which Sacks termed an "awakening." Unfortunately, this dramatic improvement in health began to reverse. Sacks' book *Awakening* first appeared in 1973. By the time his revised 1982 edition was published, seventeen of his patients were dead, mainly from Parkinsonism, and all had relapsed. Sacks describes the experiences of an encephalitis lethargica patient receiving high-dose L-dopa as follows: "For the first time, then, the patient on L-dopa enjoys a perfection of being, an ease of movement and feeling and thought, a harmony of relation within and without. Then his happy state—his world—starts to crack, slip, break down, and crumble; he lapses from his happy state, and moves toward perversion and decay."[72] Foster and Hoffer suggested that the initial improvement arose from the beneficial effect of the L-dopa and the final deleterious effect from the formation of dopachrome. The side effects of L-dopa probably come from excess formation of dopachrome-caused psychosis. A deficiency of dopamine and of dopachrome could be a factor in allowing the amyloid fibrils to develop and increased dopachrome- with adequate niacin would be therapeutic. The side effects can be avoided by giving these patients niacin in adequate doses.

It is also possible that L-dopa could be beneficial for Alzheimer's disease. I am not aware of any controlled trials treating Alzheimer's disease with L-dopa.

Foster and Hoffer[73] explain that hyperoxidation of dopamine and adrenaline is part of the cause of Parkinson's disease, multiple sclerosis, ALS, and schizophrenia. They recommend high-dose treatment with selenium, cysteine, tryptophan, and glutamine, because these nutrients are needed to make glutathione peroxidase in the body. They also recommend thiamine, riboflavin, niacin, and coenzyme Q_{10}, vitamin C, and vitamin E. Natural thyroid extract and EPA (eicosapentaenoic acid, an omega-3 fatty acid) may be beneficial, especially to schizophrenics.

Pemphigus

Pemphigus is a rare autoimmune disease that causes blisters on the skin and mucous membranes. One person suffered so horribly from pemphigus that he discovered his own cure. He had been given the best palliative treatment available, which kept him alive until he was able to create the program that has made him well for the past ten years. This is such an important case history that I (AH) am reproducing the entire letter which was submitted to the *Journal of Orthomolecular Medicine* in 2008.

> I came down with my first symptoms of pemphigus in November, 1994, just two weeks before Thanksgiving. I didn't know it at the time, because it started out as a sore throat, but by Thanksgiving Day, my mouth had begun to fill with blisters and raw spots that were so widespread and painful that I was unable to eat anything solid.
>
> After a biopsy and consultations with several specialists, I was diagnosed a month or so later with pemphigus vulgaris, a variation of pemphigus that mainly affects the mucous membranes. I came under the care of a dermatologist who would guide me through the next three years of my life, treating me for what turned out to be a very painful and stubborn disease. His first step was to put me on 20 mg of prednisone, and 100 mg of Dapsone, per day. That turned out to be much too conservative, and did nothing to relieve the pain or stop the blisters from spreading. It got to the point where I stopped eating solid food altogether, and could only tolerate bland, liquid formulas, soups, baby food, and occasionally, a cup of yogurt.
>
> By the end of March, 1995, my body and mind were so exhausted from dealing with the pain, going without food, and being unable to sleep, that I was losing hope of ever getting back to normal again. I had become delusional, thinking that my body was filled with poisons or toxins that needed to be eliminated, and I tried fasting as a last resort. That only made things worse. I had already lost forty-one pounds, and was so malnourished I could barely get out of bed, and spent the better part of the next two weeks curled up in a fetal position, trying to get comfortable, and getting up only to go to the bathroom, take a shower, or to join my family at night. There were brief moments, lying alone, when I felt as if I was leaving my body. I had

a near-death experience as a child, and again as a young adult, so I knew that feeling. I was letting go, and drifting into another world, and I didn't care. In fact, I think I would have welcomed the relief from the pain, and the sense of peace that was coming over me.

My wife had become so alarmed at my condition that she and my sister contacted the dermatologist and insisted that I be hospitalized. He hadn't seen me for over a month, and wasn't aware of how far I had slipped. He agreed to admit me to the dermatology unit at Yale-New Haven Hospital, where I was put on 80 mg of prednisone, 100 mg of Imuran, Percodan and a time-release morphine capsule, MS Contin, for pain. Because these drugs can cause debilitating side effects in themselves, I was also put on Compazine for nausea, Carafate to prevent stomach ulcers, an antibacterial rinse, stool softeners and laxatives to prevent constipation, and told to "swish and spit" with Lidocaine before each meal. Within three days, I was strong enough to go home, hopeful that my life would turn around again, but it would be several years before I was finally able to get control of my symptoms and enter into what is now a ten-year remission.

After I was released from the hospital, my treatment plan called for me to continue taking prednisone, at 80 mg, until new blisters stopped forming, and then to taper it down very slowly, in increments of 10–20 mg every other month. Each time I tried, I flared up again. Over the next two years, I was not able to get below 20 mg, and it seemed like I was always in pain, and still having difficulty eating and sleeping. The side effects of the drugs had begun to take their toll, and it felt as if I had lost my "sixth sense," and didn't know how to take what people were saying. I didn't understand the subtleties of what was being said, and had lost my ability to read between the lines, or to intuitively know when people were joking, for example, or when they were serious. I became depressed and angry, and during the worst moments, considered my situation hopeless and not worth living for. But there were also times when the higher doses of prednisone would have the opposite effect, and I would feel elated, and extremely happy with my life and my surroundings, even though the burning sensation inside my mouth was a constant reminder that I was still very sick.

Back in the 70s, I had worked as a clinical psychologist in an adolescent treatment program. My specialty was childhood schizophrenia, and I became very interested in the theories of Dr. Abram Hoffer, and Dr. Humphrey Osmond, two psychiatrists who were experimenting with the use of vitamin B_3 to treat schizophrenia.

When we are faced with a stressful situation, adrenaline is released, causing a "fight or flight" response. The source of the stress does not have to be a physical danger. It can be something as simple as a heavy work schedule, lack of sleep, or anything that touches our fears, and can become "chronic stress" when it occurs on a daily basis. Over the years, chronic stress can lead to an automatic response beyond our control, and serious psychological and physical disorders can occur. When faced with a stressful situation, we either fight back, identify the source of our stress, and stand up to it, or we turn inward, run away, and put off dealing with it to another day. Whatever our response, it is almost always accompanied by the sudden or prolonged release of adrenaline. In the case of schizophrenics, the adrenaline released under stress converts to adrenochrome, which is known to cause hallucinations. Since schizophrenia is considered to be a perceptual disorder, in that the schizophrenic "sees things" that are not there (hallucinations), and believes things that are not true (delusions), Hoffer and Osmond searched for a natural compound that would interfere with the production of adrenochrome. Dr. Hoffer, who is not only a medical doctor trained in psychiatry, but also a biochemist, knew that niacinamide is capable of blocking the conversion of adrenaline to adrenachrome. He and Dr. Humphry began administering large doses of B_3 to their patients in Saskatchewan, with great success.

I was surprised to find that one of the treatment programs for pemphigus also also involves the use of niacinamide. Usually, 500–1,000 mg of niacinamide is prescribed, 3 x day, along with an antibiotic from the tetracycline family. It is always the amide form of niacin that is used. Since pemphigus is often referred to as "a stress-related" illness, could it be that the release of adrenaline in our situation is also converted to adrenochrome, or a similar compound, causing the immune system to "see things," and to attack healthy tissues and cells?

By 1997, after two years of living with pemphigus, I was determined to get back on my feet again, and willing to try *anything*. I knew that I needed prednisone and Imuran, and followed my doctor's orders to a 'T,' but I was also hoping to find something to add to my routine that might improve my overall health, and help to put this disease behind me. I remembered what I had learned as a psychologist, and how I had experimented with Hoffer and Osmond's vitamins myself, twenty-five years earlier. I had taken up to 1,000 mg of niacinamide, the same amount of C, 100 mg of B_1, 100 mg of B_6, and 200 IU of E, 3 times a day for years, just to see how it would effect me. In general, I felt much stronger and more energetic on the vitamins than I did when I would go off of them, but the major benefit, as far as I could tell, was that I seemed to think more clearly, as if the oxygen I was breathing was going straight to my brain. If I hadn't experimented on my own, back in the 70s, I might not have thought to go back on the vitamins when I had pemphigus. Knowing they couldn't hurt me, were not contraindicated by either prednisone or Imuran, I started taking large doses of niacinamide again, along with C and the other vitamins, and waited for a miracle.

After several months, I did feel stronger again, and my appetite came back, but my blisters were no better than when I had started, and I wasn't feeling the kind of changes I had expected. I began to research the healing process in general, and discovered that zinc was used by many burn units across the country to treat severe burn injuries, and also to speed the healing of open wounds. It seemed to me that the blisters in my mouth were very much like burns (it was the same kind of pain), and were definitely open wounds, since they never seemed to heal. Adding zinc to my vitamin routine seemed like a logical approach to treating pemphigus, so I bought a bottle of Solgar's "zinc 22," and began experimenting again.

When I was younger, I was in the habit of writing in a journal, so by the end of 1997, I ended up with a very detailed account of my experience with pemphigus up to that point. I had written about the usual things, how I was feeling, what was going on around me, and my thoughts about life in general, but I had also listed all of my medications, and any changes that my doctor made to my overall treatment plan, as well as how I was feeling and whether or not I was improving from day-to-day. In the process of trying to find something that worked, I bounced back and forth between adding zinc to my diet, taking the vitamins just by themselves, or going without anything at all, but I always noted these changes as well. It wasn't until I started reading back through my journals that I saw a definite pattern: when I had added zinc at 22 mg to my diet consistently for three to four

weeks, my notes were always upbeat and positive. All of the improvements seemed to come after taking the vitamins and zinc together, so
I decided to stick to that routine. After three months, I could see the
sores in my mouth beginning to heal. I would examine them with a
flashlight as often as possible, and noticed that they were surrounded
by a ring of white tissue that seemed to be closing in on them. As the
weeks went by, the redness at the center of each lesion eventually gave
way, and only the white tissue remained. Within a week, it would turn
a healthy pink. I was also aware that pemphigus was on its way out
of my body, following the same path it had taken, but in reverse. In
other words, the most recent sores were the first to heal, followed by
the older lesions. By the end of the next three months, everything
seemed to be under control again. Not coincidentally, I had also man-
aged to taper down to 5 mg of prednisone, and went off of it completely in January, 1998. I have not had a single blister since then,
except for a brief flare-up in February of that year that lasted less than
three weeks, and after ten years of relatively perfect health, I consider
myself cured. I don't think it was merely the supplements, but on a biological level, I think they helped me to relax and to be able to better
cope with having a major illness, and the everyday ups and downs of
life that all people experience. From there, I was able to make some
major changes in my life, end a very stressful relationship, and move
further away from what I saw as the causes of my illness—without the
need for supplements or medications of any sort.

Post-Traumatic Stress Disorder

Serious though it certainly is, I (AH) do not accept Post-Traumatic Stress
Disorder (PTSD) as a legitimate psychiatric disorder. In common with all
psychiatric disorders, it is merely a description of what happens to some
people who have been subjected to enormous stress for a short period of
time or over a much longer period. The Canadian Hong Kong veterans discussed earlier in this book could be diagnosed as PTSD. Treatment of
PTSD must remove the biochemical disturbances caused by the stress.
Orthomolecular treatment is the best for this condition. One of the major
nutrients needed by these patients is niacin. The veterans were made niacin
dependent by their experiences. The stress caused sustained cellular damage that resulted in a sustained much-greater-than-average need for niacin.

Like with diabetes: some of the cells are gone, and for the rest of his or her life, a type 1 diabetic must have insulin.

Raynaud's Disease

Raynaud's disease causes extremities of the body to feel numb and cold. The smaller arteries to the skin are narrowed, limiting blood circulation to these areas. Niacin may help people with Raynaud's disease because it dilates small blood vessels, increasing circulation and providing a sense of warmth in the extremities. To feel the warm flush, one needs to select niacin, not niacinamide or no-flush niacin (inositol hexaniacinate), and take a sufficient quantity. The amount will vary from person to person.

Skin Conditions

Vitamins may be used to treat thermal burns, sunburns, wrinkles, pigmentation, scrapes, bug bites, and even bedsores. The benefits of niacin have been proven in numerous controlled clinical trials. The scientific literature contains at least twenty-nine reports published since 2003 that use niacin creams.[74–79]

Acne

It is interesting that skin and brain are both derived from ectodermal germinal tissue. I suspect they have the same nutrient needs. Often the appearance of a young person's skin will reveal a good deal about his or her nutritional state. Skin diseases that are vitamin B_3 responsive include acne, pemphigus , and epidermolysis bullosa.

In our book, *Orthomolecular Medicine for Everyone,* we wrote:

> Adolescent acne is one of the most common afflictions, but it is seldom the main complaint among the patients referred to me (AH). Rarely is it so severe that it is the primary concern. About thirty years ago, in Saskatoon, a sixteen-year-old boy was very depressed. His face was hideously covered with huge, irregular, red, oozing bumps and lumps, here and there infected. He told me he could no longer live with his face and that if my treatment did not help he would kill himself. He told me this very calmly and seriously, saying that the acne had ruined his social life.

I started the boy on a sugar-free diet, eliminated all milk products, and added a daily supplement program of niacin (3,000 milligrams), ascorbic acid (3,000 mg), pyridoxine (250 mg), and zinc sulfate (220 mg). One month later, his face was better: the vivid reddening had begun to recede, his face was no longer infected, and his mood was better. He told me he was no longer considering suicide. After three months, his face was almost clear. He was cheerful and had begun to resume his social activities at school and elsewhere.[80]

While this is a dramatic example, there are very few failures. I also advise people not to scrub their faces vigorously and not to squeeze or play with their faces. I will describe a few cases from a very large number whose acne was their main complaint and was associated with depression and anxiety. Most adolescents have minor degrees of acne: a few pimples on their face, shoulders, and back. They do not present it as a problem, but when questioned they admit they are concerned. In every case, their acne cleared on orthomolecular treatment.

I consider acne a symptom of a serious nutritional deficiency that has made the skin more susceptible to infections. Antibiotics can reduce the ravages of the infection but make the deficiency in the skin worse by their effect on the bacterial flora of the gastrointestinal tract. I have not seen antibiotics to be useful, but that may be because the cases who have been helped will not see me. Only the total failures of standard treatment come for help.

Susan, a mother of three children, had suffered from severe facial acne from childhood, but she had become so skillful with makeup that I was unaware of it, even though I had known her for many years. Several years ago, she complained to me about her acne and asked if nutrition and vitamins could help. I placed her on an orthomolecular program. Within six months, she was clear of acne, even though she had not responded to any previous treatment recommended to her by general practitioners and dermatologists. She remained well, but then began to deviate from this program and the acne came back. On resuming the nutritional program, the acne cleared and she has remained well.

Many years later Susan consulted with the Mayo Clinic in Rochester about another matter. They advised her to stop the niacin as it was very dangerous and would destroy the outer layers of her brain. (Doctors are so creative.) She did stop the niacin. Fortunately her acne did not recur, as she was still following her nutritional program and avoided foods she was allergic to. Parsons and his colleagues at the Mayo Clinic had shown many years earlier how safe niacin was.

> L.N., age twenty-five, could not remember when she was free of acne. Tetracycline helped, but whenever she went off it the acne recurred. She had several features indicating pyridoxine deficiency, including white areas on her nails, stretch marks on her body, and severe premenstrual depression. She was placed on a sugar-free program with niacin (100 mg three times daily), ascorbic acid (1,000 mg three times a day), pyridoxine (250 mg per day), and zinc sulfate (110 mg per day). Three months later, there was no improvement, so the niacin dose was increased to 500 mg three times per day; ascorbic acid to 2 grams three times per day; pyridoxine remained at 250 mg; and zinc sulfate was increased to 220 mg per day. I advised her to discontinue birth control medication. The acne began to improve in one week, and nine months after starting the program, she was well, and she has remained so for seven years.

Most mild to severe acne will respond to a diet that eliminates sugar and the foods that they are allergic to, supplemented by vitamins B_3 and C, pyridoxine, and zinc. However, optimum amounts, determined by varying the dose and judging the response, must be used. No one need suffer with acne or be exposed to the harmful effects of chronic use of tetracycline.

My patients who recover from their psychiatric illnesses invariably note a great improvement in their skin, while acne sufferers lose their depression and anxiety as the acne clears. There is a relationship that must account for some of the correlation. Simply being freed of acne will remove depression and anxiety. However, I have seen many whose acne was under control with antibiotics who still remained emotionally disturbed. Orthomolecular treatment removed both the acne and the need for tetracycline and the depression. Severe to moderate acne and psychiatric symptoms are both the result of malnutrition.

Psoriasis

The antipsoriatic drug monomethylfumarate is a niacin receptor agonist. An agonist encourages a response; it is the opposite of an antagonist. So, this drug triggers a response from a cell's niacin receptors. This is a component of Fumaderm, used in Germany for treating psoriasis.[81] Fumarate esters are potent agonists of nicotinic acid receptors in the Langerhans cells of skin, more active than 1,500 other substances. Tang and his colleagues suggested that these findings indicate that niacin may be valuable for treating psoriasis and multiple sclerosis. Niacin is valuable for treating MS and has been used as a component of an anti-MS regimen for many years, but it has to be used with caution in dealing with psoriasis.

Many years ago I (AH) treated a male schizophrenic patient with niacin. When he came back for a review one month later he was ecstatic. He told me that the psoriasis from which he had suffered, which covered his torso, was gone. He had not told me that he had had this skin disease. But the next patient I gave it to treat psoriasis became worse. After a few more trials it was clear that one could not treat patients with psoriasis safely with niacin. It might help but it might make them worse, and this became a contraindication. The flush is important in this situation. I tried the no-flush inositol derivative instead and while it had reduced effect, I was able to use it safely for patients who needed the niacin but also had psoriasis. Niacinamide did not have any impact on these skin lesions.

Skin Lesions

Skin lesions are the most prominent feature of typical pellagra. Pelle Agra means "dark skin" in Italian. It is usually correlated with exposure to sun, so pellagra in Siberia will not cause the same darkened symmetrical skin lesions found in pellagrins in Egypt. But other lesions are also found.

In September 2005, a sixty-year-old woman came to me (AH) complaining that she had been suffering from very serious skin lesions for the previous two and one half years. Her skin was blistered and had sores that had been coming and going all over her body. At the onset they were more common around her hips but more recently they had settled around her neck, face, and upper chest. Often these lesions became infected. She had seen at least nine dermatologists. In addition, she was just getting over shingles. Most of the pain was gone but there was residual scarring. And she had some arthritic-type pain. She was very depressed, spent the whole day crying, and could not work. The consensus diagnosis after a clinical conference of many dermatologists was that she was doing this to herself; it was factitious. This diagnosis was based simply on the fact that nothing had been helpful to her, thus proving it was a psychiatric condition. Pellagra was the last thing in their minds. Perhaps they had never heard of it.

Some of the dermatologists suspected that she was bringing this on herself by scratching excessively. She was very disturbed by this suggestion, pointing out that these lesions occurred even on parts of her body that she could not reach. She denied scratching and only applied certain essential oils very lightly to her lesions. In April 2005 her general practitioner, who referred her to me, received the following letter after she had been seen at a clinic:

> There was consensus of opinion, agreeing with my clinical impression of a compulsive disorder manifesting as multiple neurotic excoriations. In fact the lesions are more of a picked or pinched nature rather the frank excoriations. No one felt that any further skin biopsies or other investigations were warranted. In addition, no one felt that this was a manifestation of a paraneoplastic syndrome, as I understand that she had had abdominal or pelvic ultrasound. Her husband J. was in attendance today and I reviewed the summary and discussed the fact that there is a vicious cycle of picking at the skin and the importance of trying to break this cycle. I have also started her on Luvox 50 mg for the first week and 100 mg thereafter.

Her referring doctors noted on his referral application to me, "Numerous dermatologists feel this is a self induced rash from excoriation. I have difficulty with this."

She was aware that she was allergic to many foods and was on a dairy-free diet, as dairy products caused gas, bloating, and cramps. A rice diet for two weeks was not helpful.

The patient was a research chemist for twenty-five years and a very good observer and reporter. Serious efforts were made to help her beginning in 2003. Her medication history is very complex. Here is her account of the medication she was prescribed:

❏ December 2003: Antibiotics, prednisone, and methamethasone, hydro - val, and fucidinII.

❏ January to April 2004: 1% HC+glycerine glaxal base, bactroban/ desonide.

❏ May 2004: Suspected pemphigus. Biopsy report inconclusive.

❏ July 2004: Doxepine 10 mg, noritate cream, severe Migraine on doxepin. Prednisone added. This made the lesions worse and infections developed. Sores still present after three months.

❏ September 2004: Severe, painful lesions. Synthroid given.

❏ November 2004: Seroquel 25 mg. Appeared better on prednisone, dose increased to 50 mg.

❏ December 2004: More lesions, prednisone tapered off. Paxil started.

❏ January 2005: Celexa 20 mg started.

❏ March 2005: Discontinued Celexa.

❏ April 2005: Severe pain in three lesions on infected left inside ankle. Itching over whole body. Started tetracycline and atarax. Now had been seen by eight dermatologists. Some were concerned the lesions were self inflicted.

❏ May 2005: Completed two weeks of tetracycline. Lesions no better. All painful and wet.

❏ June 2005: Started oxycodone 5 mg for pain.

❏ July 2005: Started clindamycin 300 mg three times daily (tid).

❏ August 2005: Severe post-shingles pain in left buttock, spreading to side of thigh and leg. Given neurontin 100 mg and increased to 300 mg.

❏ September 2005: Some lesions were healing but in many areas they kept repeating, on ears, side, and back of neck, upper and lower back. Very dense around spine and thighs. Also lesions and large bumps in hair.

In addition to the prescribed medications she had been taking a large number of vitamin tablets, each containing very little vitamin.

When she came to me in September 2005 I started her on niacinamide 500 mg tid, ascorbic acid 500mg tid, l lysine 2 grams tid, zinc citrate 50 mg once daily (od); and B_{12} injections 1 mg daily, until the pain was gone.

Many physicians offer their patients large numbers of vitamin pills that contain little more of the supplement than can be found in food. These very seldom do any good. It is important to use only those few vitamins that the patients need and to allow the remainder to be obtained from their food. I used niacinamide because this patient's lesions reminded me of the lesions of pellagra. Pellagra is so rare that very few dermatologists ever think of it.

This was the second patient I encountered with pellagrous skin lesions. That first patient had seen twelve dermatologists, all over North America, with no relief. As soon as she walked into my examination room I saw the typical pellagrous lesion. A few months later, with the addition of vitamin B_3, she was well.

I did not give my present patient niacin because I felt that the flush would be too uncomfortable for her. I gave her ascorbic acid because I give it to everyone. Humans cannot make this vitamin, nor can they get enough from food. We all suffer from what Irwin Stone called hypoascorbemia, a genetic disease that prevents us from converting glucose into vitamin C, as happens in almost all other animals. The combination of the amino acid L-lysine, ascorbic acid, and injections of B_{12} is a very effective treatment for the pain of shingles and seldom fails to help within a few days. I added zinc as this mineral is very essential for the integrity of the skin.

By November of 2005 this patient, who had suffered for over two years, was free of pain. The lesions were healing. She was free of all medication except the Synthroid and was getting on very well, except for one episode when she was exposed to a room that had been recently cleaned with cleaning fluid. That made the lesions temporarily worse. She was very cheerful and pleased, and felt for the first time that the problem was being solved. I increased her nicotinamide to 1 gram tid. Her husband was delighted. He looked on this improvement as a miracle.

Trigeminal Neuralgia

Hoffer and Walker wrote:

> Trigeminal neuralgia (tic douloureux) is a disease which causes severe lancinating pain lasting several seconds to several minutes, which may be repeated many times for many months. It is often set off by touching a trigger point, or by an activity such as chewing or brushing one's teeth. The usual treatment consists of drugs such as Tegretol,

Baclofen, Phenytoin, and antidepressants, and has included surgery to sever the fifth nerve. But there is an alternative which has worked very well for four of my patients who followed it.

September 15, 1992, a woman born in 1915 told me that she had been awakened one night in 1978, screaming from pain on the right side of her face. She suffered over six episodes of severe pain. She was diagnosed tic douloureux. Since then she had not been free of pain. In addition, over the previous year she also developed severe pain in her jaw diagnosed arthritis.

I advised her to take niacin 500 mg after each meal, ascorbic acid 1,000 mg after each meal, B-complex 50s once a day, vitamin E 800 IU daily, vitamin B_{12} sublingually 2 mg per day, and folic acid 5 mg twice a day.

One week later she was free of pain. September 20, 1994, she called me to discuss something not related to this problem. I asked her about the pain. She replied it was a miracle, and she had not suffered any further pain.[82]

Niacin was a component of the treatment program for my four cases of trigeminal neuralgia, but I also advised them to take vitamin B_{12} by injection, ascorbic acid, and more lately the amino acid L-lysine. I have seen no failures with this program.

Viral Illnesses

Niacin and other B vitamins have supportive value in the treatment of viral illnesses as serious as AIDS (acquired immune deficiency syndrome). Their role may extend to having actual antiviral properties of their own. For example, thiamine (vitamin B_1) seems to have benefits for persons with chronic hepatitis B infection.[83] Additionally, a form of thiamine known as thiamine disulfide may be important for AIDS chemotherapy.[84]

Niacin deficiency is a hindrance to recovery from serious viral infection. According to Murray, "findings consistent with niacin depletion have been described in patients with AIDS. There are also clinical and laboratory data to support the potential benefit of niacin in HIV infection."[85]

Niacin would likely work best in concert with other nutrients. A 1993 Johns Hopkins study of 281 HIV-positive men showed that those taking larger-than-RDA quantities of multiple vitamin supplements had only about one-half as many new AIDS outbreaks as those not taking supplements. This important seven-year-long study has received very little publicity. That is odd, since a 50 percent reduction in AIDS cases just from vitamins should be front-page news. The real wonder is that the dosages that achieved this success were fairly small: only about five times the US RDA of the B-vitamins, vitamin C, and beta-carotene. The authors concluded that "The highest levels of total intake (from food and supplements) of vitamins C and B$_1$ and niacin were associated with a significantly decreased progression rate to AIDS (as were) vitamin A, niacin, and zinc."[86]

A 2004 Harvard study by Fawzi and colleagues also found that vitamins slow the progression to AIDS by 50 percent. In addition, vitamin supplementation cut AIDS deaths by 27 percent. The authors wrote, "Multivitamins also resulted in significantly higher CD4+ and CD8+ cell counts and significantly lower viral loads. . . . Multivitamin supplements delay the progression of HIV disease."[87]

Vitamins tend to work synergistically with each other and with other nutrients, including amino acids and minerals. This is rightfully a topic for another book, and that book has been written. *What Really Causes AIDS*[88] provides an original theory for the nutrition-based treatment of AIDS. Harry D. Foster noted highly significant nutrient deficiencies in AIDS patients, which would be more correct to describe as nutrient dependencies. The human immunodeficiency virus (HIV) is something of a biochemical parasite, which seems to fatally drain nutrients from people who are already malnourished. Dr. Foster's treatment protocol consists of supplementation with the trace mineral selenium, plus the amino acids cysteine, glutamine, and tryptophan.[89] This approach has been successfully clinically tested in South Africa, Zambia, and Uganda.[90]

Conclusion

Have no respect for the authority of others,
for there are always contrary authorities to be found.
—BERTRAND RUSSELL

Niacin, and niacin deficiency, have always been with us. The niacin molecule itself was unknown before University of Wisconsin Professor Conrad Elvehjem identified it in 1937. One may marvel at how very far we have come in understanding it in fewer than eighty years. Yet it is surprising how many physicians (not to mention pharmacists, nurses, dieticians, news reporters, and government policy makers) still insist that we don't need any more than 16 milligrams a day. (Okay, pregnant women are "allowed" a whopping 18 mg.) The RDA (Recommended Dietary Allowance) is one or even two orders of magnitude short of the optimal intake level for this very important nutrient. It is our contention that everyone needs at least several hundred mg of niacin every day. Diet cannot supply this amount. Many, perhaps most, adults probably need closer to 1,600 to 1,800 mg per day to maintain good health, and more for a therapeutic effect during illness. This is literally 100 times the RDA. Clearly, supplementation is essential.

Opposition to such dosage is strong. Hamstrung by an arbitrary but authoritative-sounding "Tolerable (or Safe) Upper Limit" of a ridiculous 35 mg per day, the vitamin-taking public has to overcome entrenched institutional bias. Long has it been said that it's not what we don't know that harms us; it's what we do know that ain't so. Never have truer words been spoken.

Niacin dosage and niacin's utility are areas of medicine where we are far from agreement with authorities. Odd, really, since high doses of niacin have been used to relieve arthritis since the 1930s. Dr. Hoffer and many medical colleagues alleviated or even cured mental illness, including schizophrenia, confusion, and learning disorders since the early 1950s. That high niacin doses are extremely effective in lowering cholesterol has been known nearly as long.

All this has led to something of a vitamin public relations problem. When vitamins are versatile, they are characterized as "faddish" and "cures in search of a disease." When pharmaceuticals are versatile, they are called "broad spectrum" and "wonder drugs." Such a double-standard needs to be exposed and opposed at every turn. We hope this book will help do so. It is high time.

Hyperactivity is not due to Ritalin deficiency, nor is high cholesterol due to a deficiency of statins, nor is arthritis caused by a deficiency of aspirin. But these seemingly unrelated health problems, and many others, may indeed be largely due to a common nutritional dependency. Treating accordingly was a good idea over half a century ago, and it is just as good today.

The Introduction of Niacin as the First Successful Treatment for Cholesterol Control

William B. Parsons, Jr., M.D., FACP (1924–2010)

My years of training in internal medicine were at the Mayo Clinic in Rochester, Minnesota. I was serving as first assistant on the Peripheral Vascular Service at St. Mary's Hospital for the summer quarter of 1955 when a series of incredible coincidences culminated in an event that changed my life. No one had any way of knowing at the time, but it also changed millions of lives around the world.

One morning, a knock interrupted our discussion in the conference room. Dr. Howard Rome, chief of the Section on Psychiatry at the Clinic, brought a surprising question: Would you be interested in hearing about a drug that reduces cholesterol levels? Skeptically (because there had been no successful drugs until then), we said that we would, of course, if there were such a drug. My mind quickly sorted through the short list of drugs that had been tried for this purpose. Thyroid had been tried but hadn't worked. Another agent that had also failed was a vegetable oil product, sitosterol, which one pharmaceutical company had marketed. I could think of no others.

The name of the drug surprised us, as Dr. Rome provided the few details he had. The preceding evening he had had dinner with Dr. Abram Hoffer, a psychiatrist from Regina, Saskatchewan, who had been in Rochester to give a series of lectures on schizophrenia. For years, he told Dr. Rome, he had administered large doses of niacin (then often called nicotinic acid) to his schizophrenic patients, feeling that it had helped them. Learning of this, his former anatomy professor at University of Saskatchewan, Dr. Rudolf Altschul, had suggested that he measure cholesterol levels in patients receiving niacin. Altschul, who had done studies of atherosclerosis in cholesterol-fed rabbits, predicted that niacin would reduce cholesterol levels. When his prediction proved correct, the two teamed with laboratory director Dr. James Stephen to try the drug in other volunteers. Their brief observations showed that niacin did, in fact, reduce cholesterol levels in a short period of time.

Early Niacin Use

Niacin was originally known as a member of the vitamin B complex, which prevents the vitamin deficiency disease pellagra in humans and black tongue in dogs. It was in all the pharmacology textbooks and well-known to doctors. Niacin was notable mainly because its administration, usually in 50 mg to 100 mg doses, was rapidly followed by flushing of the skin (redness of the skin of the face and neck, sometimes the whole upper body), accompanied by a very warm feeling, often with itching. For this reason, in vitamin preparations the closely related compound niacinamide (nicotinamide) was used because it had the vitamin activity without the flush. At that time niacin had practically no use in medicine other than its vitamin activity.

Otolaryngologists sometimes recommended it for vertigo. Physicians sometimes hoped it might help patients who had experienced a thrombotic stroke. Mayo neurologists had studied this use, along with other agents alleged to dilate intracerebral blood vessels, but found that there was really no benefit. They acknowledged that the flush might make the family think that something was being done, although there was little that could be done for a stroke in those days. The fact that it was very safe seemed to justify its use, albeit as a placebo in those instances.

Niacin was made in 50 mg or 100 mg tablets. Our first thought was that the doses used by the Canadians, 1,000 mg three or four times a day, would cause greater, intolerable flushing. Dr. Rome hastened to assure us that, according to Dr. Hoffer, flushing usually subsided in about three to four days and was no worse than with small doses. The Canadians had also briefly tried giving niacinamide. Although it caused no flush, it had failed to reduce cholesterol levels. Dr. Rome really had no further details, just these few important facts Dr. Hoffer had shared with him. It was evident that the Canadian originators had not performed a systematic trial to begin developing a useful method of treatment. Their specialties—psychiatry, anatomy, laboratory science—were not conducive to a clinical trial. On rounds that morning, I told Dr. Allen that although it sounded like a strange idea, we could easily test the claim that large doses of niacin could reduce cholesterol. In those days we did not have today's vascular surgery, which can sometimes bypass occluded leg arteries. Therefore we kept numerous patients in the hospital for weeks while we did everything medically possible to increase circulation, trying to heal ulcers on feet or legs. If our efforts failed and the leg became gangrenous, amputation was usually necessary, frequently above the knee. With so much at stake we often lavished weeks of hospital care, attempting to save a limb. One must remember that hospital charges at that time were reasonable.

Niacin/Cholesterol Trials

We customarily measured cholesterol and other blood lipids as part of our admission workup, even though we had no good method for improving abnormal lipids beyond altering diet. Then, as now, diet was a weak and often ineffective way to reduce elevated cholesterol levels. I told Dr. Allen that I could recheck lipids on five or six patients with hypercholesteremia, tell them about the new treatment, and see whether we could verify the Canadian observations. Dr. Allen gave his blessing and promptly forgot about it. I have always been grateful for his approval.

I found five patients on the service with high cholesterol levels and a vascular status that would keep them hospitalized for several weeks. That afternoon, at the bedside of each patient, I recited the fragmentary word-of-mouth report we had received and invited them to take part in a brief trial of a well-known drug, widely regarded as safe, to see whether it really did reduce cholesterol. I described the flush and assured them it would subside in a few days if our informant had been correct.

The patients agreed and began taking tablets (ten 100 mg tablets with each meal), after another baseline blood test. The flush lessened and disappeared in the first week, as predicted. So far, so good. After one week I repeated the lipid studies and could not believe the striking reductions in cholesterol, triglycerides, and total lipids. In disbelief, I waited for the second week's results (as good or better) before showing the results to the others on the service. The initial hospital trial continued for four weeks, by which time it was apparent that a longer, carefully planned study was the next step.

The Mayo Clinic has a section just for care of Rochester residents. One of the young consultants in that section was my close friend, Dr. Richard Achor. He and Dr. Kenneth Berge (whom I hadn't met until then because he joined the staff during my two-year absence) had a list of patients with hypercholesteremia, which they gave me to recruit volunteers. By telephone I obtained eighteen participants for at least twelve weeks of study, using niacin in 1,000 mg doses with meals and measuring cholesterol weekly.

Laboratory scientist Dr. Bernard McKenzie brought a unique contribution to the study. His laboratory had been separating cholesterol fractions by electrophoresis, giving us a means of determining beta-lipoprotein cholesterol (now LDL cholesterol) and alpha1-lipoprotein cholesterol (now HDL cholesterol). Preliminary studies had shown that a high ratio of beta to alpha 1 cholesterol often led to premature heart attacks. We incorporated his testing into our study.

The results were just as impressive as in the preliminary hospital observations. There were marked cholesterol reductions in the first week in many, if not most, participants. Not only that, but the cholesterol fraction was the site of major reduction, accompanied by an increase in the fraction.

My Mayo colleagues encouraged me to report this promising new treatment before leaving Rochester in April 1956 to practice with a Madison, Wisconsin clinic. The paper I presented at a staff meeting was published in June in the *Proceedings of the Staff Meetings of the Mayo Clinic*,[1] the prestigious journal with world-wide circulation which since then has shortened its name to *Mayo Staff Proceedings*.

At the time I realized that I was reporting the first successful cholesterol-lowering drug in history. My enthusiasm was tempered by the knowledge that it would have to be studied in many persons for years just to show that it remained effective, that it was safe in prolonged use, and that reducing cholesterol would, as we hoped, reduce atherosclerosis and prevent its disastrous complications.

The Mayo publication was important because it reported to its wide circulation the first systematic study, including the favorable results in the cholesterol fractions. Altschul, Hoffer, and Stephen had earlier published a letter to the editor of the *Archives of Biochemistry and Biophysics*[2] which might have been overlooked by clinical investigators and never implemented.

I first presented the updated Mayo report at the November 1956 meeting of the *American Society for the Study of Arteriosclerosis,* its first airing at a national meeting. (The ASSA later became the Council on Arteriosclerosis of the American Heart Association.) I first met Dr. Rudolf Altschul at their November 1957 meeting, saw him at any subsequent ASSA meetings he attended, and contributed a chapter to his book[3] on what was then known about niacin, which he was editing when he died in 1963. Of current interest, I recall his talk at the 1957 or 1958 meeting about his rabbit work, in which he showed that niacin strikingly reduced the foam cell content of atherosclerotic plaques. This is now especially significant in view of emphasis in recent years on rupture-prone plaques as a cause of sudden arterial occlusion, even when the narrowing is no more than 50 percent of the arterial diameter.

I had never met Abram Hoffer when, in 1990, we had a momentous telephone conversation, which convinced me more than ever about my meant-to-be hypothesis. The story of how niacin came to be tested in hypercholesteremia was stranger than I had expected. In 1952 Hoffer had experienced some bleeding from the gums, for which he had taken vitamin C without benefit. He had already been using niacin for schizophrenic patients and decided to take three grams daily to see how the flush felt. His gums improved. He reasoned that niacin had promoted rapid healing in gums which had been affected by chronic malocclusion and, with age, had not been healing as well as in earlier years.

Dr. Hoffer's use of niacin in schizophrenia began in 1952, at which time he was using three to six grams per day, as well as niacinamide. He called his work the first double-blind psychiatric study ever performed. In the mid-1950s he lived and practiced in Regina. Dr. Altschul, who had been Hoffer's professor of anatomy in medical school at Saskatoon, had been doing oxidation experiments, exposing rabbits to ultraviolet light and to increased concentrations of oxygen in inspired air to see whether these measures would somehow alter cholesterol deposition in arteries.

On one occasion Professor Altschul sought to arrange a trial in humans for his idea that exposure to ultraviolet light might reduce cholesterol levels. He contacted his former student, Abram Hoffer, who was Director of Research for the province, and asked for his help in setting up such a study at Saskatchewan Hospital, a 1,600-bed mental hospital in Wayburn. They planned a joint visit to the hospital for this purpose. Dr. Altschul took a train to Regina, and together they drove to Wayburn, seventy-one miles away.

During the drive they talked about their individual interests. Altschul expressed his opinion that atherosclerotic plaques developed because of injury to the intima. He went on to speculate that the intima was not healing fast enough. Hoffer suggested a trial of niacin, based on his personal experience with bleeding gums.

In our telephone conversation, Hoffer told me that when he made his suggestion, Dr. Altschul didn't know what niacin was! Having received large quantities of niacin and niacinamide for his work, Hoffer gave a pound of niacin powder (about 450 grams) to his former anatomy professor, who then fed it to rabbits whose blood cholesterol had been elevated to very high levels by dietary maneuvers well-known to animal researchers. How he knew how much niacin to use is among the bits of information still lacking, but apparently niacin reduced the blood cholesterol levels within days. Hoffer reported that Altschul then phoned him, excitedly shouting, "It works! It works!"

Until that September 1990 conversation, I had never known who Jim Stephen was. Hoffer explained that he was the chief pathologist and laboratory director at the hospital in Regina where Hoffer practiced.

With his permission, in 1954 Hoffer did a two-day study, giving niacin to about sixty patients who demonstrated a reduction in their cholesterol levels. Altschul, Hoffer, and Stephen then wrote their letter to the editor of *Archives of Biochemistry and Biophysics*.[4]

In our phone conversation, I picked up the story and told Hoffer of the chain of events which had brought his information to me and resulted in my decision to do further studies. He had never before heard the details. He had many complimentary comments about my research in the following years, correctly recognizing that it had provided the impetus that resulted in niacin's becoming a major cholesterol-control agent. We closed our telephone conversation with the mutual wish that we might some day get together to discuss our shared interests face-to-face.

In the fall of 1997, a medical association in Victoria to which Dr. Hoffer belongs invited me to speak to them and the public about my work with niacin and my book, *Cholesterol Control Without Diet! The Niacin Solution*.[5] This was the pilgrimage I had always envisioned to meet Dr. Hoffer. We used it for a dual purpose, which included beginning the promotion for the book. I finally met Abram Hoffer in person for the first time in the driveway of the Empress Hotel in Victoria, on November 11, 1998, more than forty-three years after my first use of niacin for hypercholesteremia. It was his eightieth birthday.

We reviewed the circumstances that had brought us together and all that niacin had come to mean to doctors and their patients around the world. We hoped that my book would teach patients the importance of niacin's distinctive advantages, not shared by any other cholesterol-control drugs, and also show doctors how to become proficient at using niacin.

I have always been happy to share with the Canadian originators whatever credit there may be for pioneering the use of niacin for cholesterol control and for its eventual reduction of heart attacks (24 percent), strokes (26 percent), cardiovascular surgery (46 percent), and deaths (11 percent, adding a mean of 1.63 years of life to men 30 to 65 years old with one or more preceding heart attacks).[6] Without their vision and Hoffer's taking their observations to the Mayo Clinic, I would not have been able to perform the first systematic study and follow it with further research in Madison, leading to the Coronary Drug Project's demonstration of niacin's preventive effects in cardiovascular disease.[7] Dr. Hoffer has correctly said that while pioneers in many fields argue about precedence, we are friends who readily acknowledge each other's roles in starting niacin research. Clearly, it was meant to be.

(Abridged and reprinted with permission of the *Journal of Orthomolecular Medicine*, 2000. 15:3. Footnotes renumbered.)

References

Foreword

1. Brown, G. B. "Niaspan in the Management of Dyslipidaemia: The Evidence." *Eur Heart J Suppl* 8 (2006): F60-F67.

2. Villines, T. C., E. J. Stanek, P. J. Devine, et al. "The ARBITER 6-HALTS Trial (Arterial Biology for the Investigation of the Treatment Effects of Reducing Cholesterol 6-HDL and LDL Treatment Strategies in Atherosclerosis): Final Results and the Impact of Medication Adherence, Dose, and Treatment Duration." *J Am Coll Cardiol* 55 (2010): 2721–2726.

3. Coleman, M. "Axon Degeneration Mechanisms: Commonality Amid Diversity." *Nat Rev Neurosci* 6 (2005): 889–898.

4. Adalbert, R., T. H. Gillingwater, J. E. Haley, et al. "A Rat Model of Slow Wallerian Degeneration (WldS) with Improved Preservation of Neuromuscular Synapses." *Eur J Neurosci* 21, (2005): 271–277.

5. Araki, T., Y. Sasaki, J. Milbrandt. "Increased Nuclear NAD Biosynthesis and SIRT1 Activation Prevent Axonal Degeneration." *Science* 305 (2004): 1010–1013.

6. Ibid.

7. Penberthy, W. T., and I. Tsunoda. "The Importance of NAD in Multiple Sclerosis." *Curr Pharm Des* 15 (2009): 64–99.

8. Lin, S. J., P. A. Defossez, L. Guarente. "Requirement of NAD and SIR2 for Lifespan Extension by Calorie Restriction in Saccharomyces Cerevisiae." *Science* 289 (2000): 2126–2128.

9. Penberthy, W. Todd, Kristian B. Axelsen. "Table of NAD-Utilizing Enzymes," http://web.me.com/wtpenber/NAD-Utilizing_Enzymes/1.html

Introduction: Why Should You Read This Book?

1. Kuhn, T. S. *The Structure of Scientific Revolutions.* Chicago, IL: Chicago University Press, 1962.

2. Moore, T. J. *Deadly Medicine: Why Tens of Thousands of Heart Patients Died in America's Worst Drug Disaster.* New York, NY: Simon and Schuster, 1995.

3. Abramson, J. *Overdo$ed America: The Broken Promise of American Medicine.* New York, NY: Harper Perennial, 2005.

4. Dean, C., T. Tuck. *Death by Modern Medicine.* Belleville, ON: Matrix Vérité Media, 2005.

5. Pauling, L. *How to Live Longer and Feel Better.* New York, NY: W.H. Freeman, 1986.

6. Pauling, L. "Orthomolecular Psychiatry." *Science* 160 (1968): 265–271.

7. Hoffer, A., A. W. Saul. *Orthomolecular Medicine for Everyone: Megavitamin Therapeutics for Families and Physicians.* Laguna Beach, CA: Basic Health Publications, 2008.

8. Ibid.

9. Ibid.

10. Williams, R. *Biochemical Individuality.* New York, NY: W. H. Freeman, 1956.

11. Foster, H. D. *Reducing Cancer Mortality: A Geographical Perspective.* Victoria, BC: Western Geographical Press, 1986.

12. Foster H. D. *What Really Causes Alzheimer's Disease.* Victoria, BC: Trafford Publishing, 2004. http://www.hdfoster.com/publications

13. University of Maryland Medical Center, *Sulfur.* http://www.umm.edu/altmed/articles/sulfur-000328.htm

14. Williams, S.R. *Nutrition and Diet Therapy,* 6th ed., St. Louis, MO: Times-Mirror/Mosby, 1989: 239.

Chapter 1: What Is Niacin?

1. Gutierrez, D. "Niacin May Lower the Risk of Heart Disease." NaturalNews.com (Nov 7, 2008): http://www.naturalnews.com/024745_niacin_cholesterol_research.html

2. Penberthy, W T. "Nicotinic Acid-Mediated Activation of Both Membrane and Nuclear Receptors towards Therapeutic Glucocorticoid Mimetics for Treating Multiple Sclerosis." *PPAR Res* (2009): 853707.

3. Penberthy, W. T., I. Tsunoda. "The Importance of NAD in Multiple Sclerosis." *Curr Pharm Des* 15(1) (2009): 64–99. Review.

4. Penberthy, W. T. "Nicotinamide Adenine Dinucleotide Biology and Disease." *Curr Pharm Des* 15(1) (2009): 1–2.

5. Hoffer, A. "Patentable vs. Non-patentable Treatment," *J Orthomolecular Med* 14 (2nd Quarter 1999): Editorial.

6. Hoffer, A. "Megavitamin B_3 Therapy for Schizophrenia." *Can Psychiat Assoc J* 16 (1971): 499–504.

7. Dalton, T. A., R. S. Berry. "Hepatotoxicity Associated With Sustained-release Niacin." *Am J Med* 93(1) (Jul 1992): 102–4.

8. Guyton, J. R., H. E. Bays. "Safety Considerations With Niacin Therapy." *Am J Cardiol* 19;99(6A) (Mar 2007): 22C–31C.

9. Citations from original source:

19. Henkin, Y., A. Oberman, D. C. Hurst, et al. "Niacin Revisited: Clinical Observations on an Important But Underutilized Drug." *Am J Med* 91 (1991): 239–246.

20. Henkin, Y., K. C. Johnson, J. P. Segrest. "Rechallenge With Crystalline Niacin After Drug-induced Hepatitis From Sustained-release Niacin." *J Am Med Assoc* 264 (1990): 241–243.

3. McKenney, J. M., J. D. Proctor, S. Harris, et al. "A Comparison of the Efficacy and Toxic Effects of Sustained- Vs. Immediate-release Niacin in Hypercholesterolemic Patients." *J Am Med Assoc* 271 (1994): 672–677.

10. Loriaux, S. M., J. B. Deijen, J. F. Orlebeke, et al. "The Effects of Nicotinic Acid and Xanthinol Nicotinate on Human Memory in Different Categories of Age. A Double Blind Study." *Psychopharmacology (Berl)* 87(4) (1985): 390–5.

11. Perricone, N. V., D. Bagchi, B. Echard, et al. "Blood Pressure Lowering Effects of Niacin-bound Chromium(III) (NBC) in Sucrose-fed Rats: Renin-angiotensin System." *J Inorg Biochem102(7) (Jul 2008): 1541–8.*

12. Preuss, H. G., D. Wallerstedt, N. Talpur, et al. "Effects of Niacin-bound Chromium and Grape Seed Proanthocyanidin Extract on the Lipid Profile of Hypercholesterolemic Subjects: A Pilot Study." *J Med* 31(5–6) (2000): 227–46.

13. Preuss, H. G., B. Echard, N. V. Perricone, et al. "Comparing Metabolic Effects of Six Different Commercial Trivalent Chromium Compounds." *J Inorg Biochem* 102(11) (Nov 2008): 1986–90.

14. Preuss, H. G., S. T. Jarrell, R. Scheckenbach, et al. "Comparative Effects of Chromium, Vanadium and Gymnema Sylvestre on Sugar-induced Blood Pressure Elevations in SHR." *J Am Coll Nutr* 17(2) (Apr 1998): 116–23.

Chapter 2. How Niacin Therapy Began

1. Elmore, J. G., A. R. Feinstein. "Joseph Goldberger: An Unsung Hero of American Clinical Epidemiology." *Ann Intern Med* 121(5) (Sep 1994): 372–5.

2. National Institutes of Health, Office of History. "Dr. Joseph Goldberger & the War on Pellagra" http://history.nih.gov/exhibits/goldberger/index.html

3. Wittenborn, J. R. "A Search for Responders to Niacin Supplementation." *Arch Gen Psychiat* 31 (1974): 547–552.

Chapter 3. How Niacin Works, and Why We Need More of It

1. Merialdi, M., L. E. Caulfield, N. Zavaleta, et al. "Randomized Controlled Trial of Prenatal Zinc Supplementation and the Development of Fetal Heart Rate." *Am J Obstet Gynecol* 190 (2004): 1106–1112.

2. Wu, G., F. W. Baze, T. A. Cudd, et al. "Maternal Nutrition and Fetal Development." *J Nut* 134 (2004): 2169–2172.

3. Ibid.

4. Hetzel, B. S. *The Story of Iodine Deficiency: An International Challenge in Nutrition.* Oxford, ENG: Oxford University Press, 1989.

5. Tan, J., R. Li, W. Zhu. "Medical Geography." In: M. Ren, C. Lin, eds. *Recent Development of Geographical Science in China.* Beijing: Science Press, 1990. 259–279.

6. Ibid.

7. Wu, Baze, Cudd, et al. "Maternal Nutrition" *J Nut* 134: 2169–2172.

8. Foster, H. D., A. Hoffer. "The Two Faces of L-Dopa: Benefits and Adverse Side-effects in the Treatment of Encephalitis Lethargica, Parkinson's Disease, Multiple Sclerosis and Amyotrophic Lateral Sclerosis." *Med Hypotheses* 62(2) (2004): 177–181.

9. Foster, H. D. *What Really Causes Multiple Sclerosis.* Victoria, BC: Trafford Publishing, 2007.

10. Wu, Baze, Cudd, et al. "Maternal Nutrition" *J Nut* 134: 2169–2172.

11. Hartl, D. L., D. Freifelder, L. Synder. *Basic Genetics.* Boston, MA: Jones et Bartlett, 1988.

12. Ames, B. N., I. Elson-Schwab, E. A. Silver. "High-dose Vitamin Therapy Stimulates Variant Enzymes with Decreased Coenzyme Binding Affinity (Increased K_m): Relevance to Genetic Disease and Polymorphisms." *Am J Clin Nutr* 75 (2002): 616–658.

13. Ibid.

14. Ibid.

15. Barleer, G. W., G. L. Spaeth. "The Successful Treatment of Homocystinuria With Pyridoxine." *J Pediatr* 75 (1969): 463–478.

16. Neu, H. C. "The Crisis in Antibiotic Resistance." *Science* 257(5073) (1992): 1064–1073.

17. Foster H. D. "Host-pathogen Evolution: Implications for the Prevention and Treatment of Malaria, Myocardial Infarction and AIDS." *Med Hypotheses.* 2008; 70: 21–25.

18. Mizuno, Y., S. I. Kawazu, S. Kano, et al. "In Vitro Uptake of Vitamin A by Plasmodium Falciparum." *Ann Trop Med Parasit* 97(3) (2003): 237–243.

19. Andrews, K. T., T. N. Tran, N. C. Wheatley, et al. "Targeting Histone Deacetylase Inhibitors for Anti-malarial Therapy." *Curr Top Med Chem* 9(3) (2009): 292–308.

20. Shankar, A. H., B. Genton, R. D. Semba, et al. "Effects of Vitamin A Supplemen-

tation on Morbility Due to Plasmodium Falciparum in Young Children in Papua New Guinea: A Randomized Trial." *Lancet* 354(9174) (1999): 203–209.

21. Foster, H. D. "Coxsackie B Virus and Myocardial Infarction." *Lancet* 359(9308) (2002): 804.

22. Cermelli, C., M. Vincet, E. Scaltriti, et al. "Selenium Inhibition of Coxsackie B5 Replication on the Etiology of Keshan Disease." *J Trace Elem Med Bio* 16(1) (2002): 41–46.

23. Kuklinski, B., E. Weissenbacher, A. Fähnrich. "Coenzyme Q_{10} and Antioxidants in Acute Myocardial Infarction." *Mol Aspects Med* 15(Suppl) (1994): 143–147.

24. Foster, H. D. *What Really Causes AIDS.* Victoria, BC: Trafford Publishing, 2002. http://www.hdfoster.com/publications

25. Namulema, E., J. Sparling, H. D. Foster. "Nutritional Supplements Can Delay the Progress of AIDS in HIV-infected Patients: Results from a Double-blinded, Clinical Trial at Mengo Hospital, Kampala, Uganda." *J Orthomolecular Med* 22(3) (2007): 129–136.

26. Xu, Q., C. G. Parks, L. A. Deroo, R. M. Cawthor, et al. "Multivitamin Use and Telomere Length in Women." *Am J Clin Nutr* 89(6) (2009): 1857–1863.

27. Bize, P., F. Criscuolo, N. B. Metcalfe, et al. "Telomere Dynamics Rather Than Age Predict Life Expectancy in the Wild." *P Biol Sci/R Soc.* 276(1662) (2009): 1679–1683.

28. 7. Hoffer, A., H. D. Foster. *Feel Better, Live Longer with Vitamin B_3: Nutrient Deficiency and Dependency.* Toronto, ON: CCNM Press, 2007.

29. Miller, C.L., J. R. Dulay. "The High-affinity Niacin Receptor HM74A is Decreased in the Anterior Cingulate Cortex of Individuals with Schizophrenia." *Brain Res Bull* 77(1) (Sep 5, 2008): 33–41.

30. Horrobin, D. *The Madness of Adam and Eve. How Schizophrenia Shaped Humanity.* London, ENG: Bantam Press, 2001.

31. Huxley, J., E. Mayr, H. Osmond, A. Hoffer. "Schizophrenia as a Genetic Morphism." *Nature* 204 (1964): 220–221.

32. Foster, Hoffer. "The Two Faces of L-Dopa" *Med Hypothesis* 62: 177–181.

33. Cleave, T.L. *Diabetes, Coronary Thrombosis, and the Saccharine Disease.* Bristol, ENG: John Wright & Sons, 1966.

34. Miller, Dulay. "The High-affinity Niacin Receptor HM74A" *Brain Res Bull* 77(1): 33–41.

35. Hoffer, A., H. D. Foster. *Feel Better, Live Longer With Niacin.* Toronto, ON: CCNM Press, 2007.

36. Hawthorn, T. Obituary. *Globe and Mail* Toronto, ON: November 29, 2008

37. Green, G. "Subclinical Pellagra." In: D. Hawkins, L. Pauling, eds. *Orthomolec-*

ular Psychiatry Treatment of Schizophrenia San Francisco, CA: WH Freeman, 1973. 411–433.

38. Kaufman, W. *The Common Form of Niacin Amide Deficiency Disease: Aniacinamidosis.* New Haven, CT: Yale University Press, 1943.

39. Kaufman, W. "Niacinamide: A Most Neglected Vitamin." *J Int Acad Prev Med* 8 (1983): 5–25.

40. Miller, Dulay. "The High-affinity Niacin Receptor HM74A" *Brain Res Bull* 77(1): 33–41.

Chapter 4. How to Take Niacin

1. "Doctors Say, Raise the RDAs Now." Orthomolecular Medicine News Service, Oct 30, 2007 http://orthomolecular.org/resources/omns/v03n10.shtml7

2. Merck Manual, Online Medical Library, Home Ed. "Disorders of Nutrition and Metabolism: Vitamins." http://www.merckmanuals.com/home/sec12/ch154/ch154a.html

3. Troppmann, L., K. Gray-Donald, T. Johns. "Supplement Use: Is There Any Nutritional Benefit?" *J Am Diet Assoc* 102(6) (June 1, 2002): 818–825.

4. Ibid.

5. Passwater, R. A. *Supernutrition,* New York, NY: Pocket Books, 1991.

6. Rohte, O., D. Thormählen, P. Ochlich. ["Elucidation of the Mechanism of Nicotinic Acid Flush in Animal Experimentation."] [Article in German] *Arzneimittelforschung* 7(12) (1977): 2347–52.

7. Kunin, R. A. "Manganese and Niacin in the Treatment of Drug-induced Dyskinesias." *J Orthomol Psych,* 5(1) (1976): 4–27.

8. Kaijser, L., B. Eklund, A. G. Olsson, et al. "Dissociation of the Effects of Nicotinic Acid on Vasodilatation and Lipolysis by a Prostaglandin Synthesis Inhibitor, Indomethacin, in Man." *Med Biol* 57(2) (Apr 1979): 114–7.

9. Estep, D. L., G. R. Gay, R. T. Rappolt, Sr. "Preliminary report of the Effects of Propranolol HCl on the Discomfiture Caused by Niacin." *Clin Toxicol* 11(3) (1977): 325–8.

10. Boyle, E. "Niacin and the Heart." Paper delivered at Int. Conf. Alcoholics Anonymous Physicians, New York, 1967 (excerpted in *A Second Communication to A.A.'s Physicians,* Bedford Hills, NY: 1968).

11. Cheng, K., T. J. Wu, K. K. Wu, et al. "Antagonism of the Prostaglandin D2 Receptor 1 Suppresses Nicotinic Acid-induced Vasodilation in Mice and Humans." *P Natl Acad Sci USA.* 103(17) (Apr 25, 2006): 6682–7.

12. Bicknell, F., F. Prescott. *The Vitamins in Medicine,* 3rd ed., p 379. London, ENG: William Heinemann Medical Books Ltd, 1953. Reprint: Milwaukee, WI: Lee Foundation for Nutritional Research.

Chapter 5. Safety of Niacin

1. Vague, P. H., B. Vialtettes, V. Lassmanvague, et al. "Nicotinamide May Extend Remission Phase in Insulin Dependent Diabetes." *Lancet* 1 (1987): 619–620.

2. Canner, P. L., C. D. Furberg, M. E. McGovern. "Benefits of Niacin in Patients With Versus Without the Metabolic Syndrome and Healed Myocardial Infarction (from the Coronary Dug Project)" *Am J Cardiol* 97(4) (Feb 2006): 477–479.

3. Dube, M. P., et al. "Safety and Efficacy of Extended-release Niacin for the Treatment of Dyslipidaemia in Patients with HIV Infection: AIDS Clinical Trials Group Study A5148." *Antivir Ther* 11(8) (2006): 1081–1089.

4. Kirkey, A. "Diabetics Should Take Cholesterol-lowering Drugs, Study Finds." *Edmonton Journal* Jan 11, 2008.

5. Zhou, S. S., D. Li, W. P. Sun, et al. "Nicotinamide Overload May Play a Role in the Development of Type 2 Diabetes." *World J Gastroenterol* 15(45) (Dec 7, 2009): 5674–84.

6. Li, D., W. P. Sun, Y. M. Zhou al. "Chronic Niacin Overload May Be Involved in the Increased Prevalence of Obesity in US Children." *World J Gastroenterol* 16(19) (May 21, 2010): 2378–2387.

7. Dajani HM, Lauer AK. Optical coherence tomography findings in niacin maculopathy. *Can J Ophthalmol* 2006; 41:197–200.

8. Freisberg L, Rolle, TJ, Ip MS. Diffuse Macular Edema in Niacin-Induced Maculopathy May Resolve With Dosage Decrease. *Retinal Cases & Brief Reports* 5:227–228 doi: 10.1097/ICB.0b013e3181e180c0

9. Millay RH, Klein ML, Illingworth DR. Niacin maculopathy. *Ophthalmology* 1998; 95:930–936.

10. Fraunfelder FW, Fraunfelder FT, and Illingworth DR. Adverse ocular effects associated with niacin therapy. *Br J Ophthalmol* 1995; 79:54–56.

11. Fraunfelder FW. Ocular side effects from herbal medicines and nutritional supplements. *Amer J Ophthalmol* 2004; 138:639–647.

12. Mularski, R. A., R. E. Grazer, L. Santoni, et al. "Treatment Advice on the Internet Leads to a Life-threatening Adverse reaction: Hypotension Associated with Niacin Overdose." *Clin Toxicol (Phila)* 44(1) (2006): 81–4.

13. Bays, H. E., D. Maccubbin, A. G. Meehan, et al. "Blood Pressure-lowering Effects of Extended-release Niacin Alone and Extended-release Niacin/Laropiprant Combination: A Post Hoc Analysis of a 24-Week, Placebo-controlled Trial in Dyslipidemic Patients." *Clin Ther* (1) (Jan 2009): 115–22.

14. Bays, H. E., D. J. Rader. "Does Nicotinic acid (Niacin) Lower Blood Pressure?" *Int J Clin Pract* 63(1) (Jan 2009): 151–9.

15. Parsons, W. B. Jr. *Cholesterol Control without Diet! The Niacin Solution.* 2nd ed., Scottsdale, AZ: Lilac Press, 2003.

16. Bronstein, A. C., D. A. Spyker, L. R. Cantilena Jr., et. al. "2009 Annual Report of the American Association of Poison Control Centers' National Poison Data System (NPDS): 27th Annual Report." *Clinical Toxicology* 48 (2010): 979–1178. The data mentioned in the inset are found in Table 22B, journal pages 1138–1148.

17. Gonzalez-Heydrich, J., R. D. Wilens, A. Leichtner, et al. "Retrospective Study of Hepatic Enzyme Elevations in Children Treated with Olanzapine, Divalproic Acid and Their Combination." *J Am Acad Child Adolescent Psych* 42 (2003): 1227–33.

18. Bronstein AC, Spyker DA, Cantilena LR Jr, Green JL, Rumack BH, Giffin SL. 2009 Annual Report of the American Association of Poison Control Centers' National Poison Data System (NPDS): 27th Annual Report. Clinical Toxicology (2010). 48, 979–1178. The vitamin data mentioned in the inset are found in Table 22B.

19. Kemper, K. J., K. L. Hood. "Does Pharmaceutical Advertising Affect Journal Publication About Dietary Supplements?" *BMC Complement Altern Med* 8(11) (Apr 9, 2008). Full text at http://www.biomedcentral.com/1472–6882/8/11 or http://www.pubmedcentral.nih.gov/articlerender.fcgi?tool=pubmed&pubmedid=18400092

20. Ibid.

21. Vedantam, S. "Drug Studies Skewed Toward Study Sponsors: Industry-funded Research Often Favors Patent-holders, Study Finds." *The Washington Post*, April 11, 2006. http://www.msnbc.msn.com/id/12275329/from/RS.5/

22. Heres, S., J. Davis, K. Maino, et al. "Why Olanzapine Beats Risperidone, Risperidone Beats Quetiapine, and Quetiapine Beats Olanzapine: An Exploratory Analysis of Head-to-Head Comparison Studies of Second-Generation Antipsychotics." *Am J Psychiat* 163 (Feb 2006): 185–194. http://ajp.psychiatryonline.org/cgi/content/full/163/2/185

23. Angell, M. *The Truth about the Drug Companies*. New York, NY: Random House, 2004.

24. Ibid.

25. Vedantam. "Drug Studies Skewed Toward Study Sponsors" http://www.msnbc.msn.com/id/12275329/from/RS.5/

26. Stroup, T. S., Lieberman, J. A., J. P. McEvoy, et al. "Effectiveness of Olanzapine, Quetiapine, Risperidone, and Ziprasidone in Patients with Chronic Schizophrenia Following Discontinuation of a Previous Atypical Antipsychotic." *Am J Psychiat* 163(4) (Apr 2006): 611–22.

Chapter 6. Pandeficiency Disease

1. Marini, N. J., J. Gin, J. Ziegle, et al. "The Prevalence of Folate-remedial MTHFR Enzyme Variants in Humans." *P Natl Acad Sci USA* 105(23) (Jun 10, 2008): 8055–60.

2. Cleave, T. L. *The Saccharine Disease.* New Canaan, CT: Keats Publishing, 1975.

3. Cleave, T. L. *Diabetes, Coronary Thrombosis, and the Saccharine Disease.* Bristol, ENG: John Wright & Sons, 1966.

4. Hoffer, A., M. Walker. *Orthomolecular Nutrition.* New Canaan, CT: Keats Publishing, 1978.

5. Yudkin, J. *Sweet and Dangerous.* New York, NY: Peter H Wyden, 1972.

6. Challem, J., B. Berkson, M. D. Smith. *Syndrome X: The Complete Nutritional Program to Prevent and Reverse Insulin Resistance.* New York, NY: Wiley, 2000.

7. Marini, Gin, Ziegle, et al. "The Prevalence of Folate-remedial MTHFR" *P Natl Acad Sci USA* 105(23): 8055–60.

8. Ames, B. N., I. Elson-Schwab, E. A. Silver. "High-dose Vitamin Therapy Stimulates Variant Enzymes With Decreased Coenzyme Binding Affinity (Increased K(m)): Relevance to Genetic Disease and Polymorphisms." *Am J Clin Nutr* 75(4) (Apr 2002): 616–58.

9. Hoffer, Walker. *Orthomolecular Nutrition.*

10. USDA Economic Research Service. "U.S. Sugar Consumption Continues to Grow." *USDA Agr Outlook* (March 1997).

11. Hoffer, A., A. W. Saul. *Orthomolecular Medicine for Everyone: Megavitamin Therapeutics for Families and Physicians.* Laguna Beach, CA: Basic Health Publications, 2008.

12. Baker, S. M. "What's 'Biomedical'?" *Autism Res Rev Int* 21 (2007): 3. Guest editorial.

Chapter 7. Reversing Arthritis with Niacinamide:
The Pioneering Work of William Kaufman, M.D., Ph.D.

1. Kaufman, W. *The Common Form of Joint Dysfunction: Its Incidence and Treatment.* Brattleboro, VT: E. L. Hildreth & Company, 1949.

2. Kaufman, W. "The Use of Vitamins to Reverse Certain Concomitants of Aging." *J Am Geriatr Soc* 3 (1955): 927–936.

3. Jonas, W. B., C. P. Rapoza, W. F. Blair. "The Effect of Niacinamide in Osteoarthritis: A Pilot Study." *Inflamm Res* 45 (July 1996): 330–334.

4. Lukaczer, D., *Nutr Sci* (Nov 1999).

5. Hoffer, A. "Treatment of Arthritis by Nicotinic Acid and Nicotinamide." *Can Med Assoc J* 81 (1959): 235–238.

6. Gardiner, H., A. Berenson. "10 Voters on Panel Backing Pain Pills Had Industry Ties." *New York Times,* February 25, 2005.

7. Hoffer, A., H. D. Foster. *Feel Better, Live Longer With Vitamin B₃: Nutrient Deficiency and Dependency.* Toronto, ON: CCNM Press, 2007.

8. Psaty, B. M., Kronmal, R. A. "Reporting Mortality Findings in Trials of Rofecoxib for Alzheimer Disease or Cognitive Impairment: A Case Study Based on Documents from Rofecoxib Litigation." *J Am Med Assoc* ;299(15) (Apr 16, 2008): 1813–7.

9. Ross, J. S., K. P. Hill, D. S. Egilman, et al. "Guest Authorship and Ghostwriting in Publications Related to Rofecoxib: A Case Study of Industry Documents from Rofecoxib Litigation." *J Am Med Assoc* 299(15) (Apr 16, 2008): 1800–12.

10. DeAngelis, C. D., P. B. Fontanarosa. "Impugning the Integrity of Medical Science: The Adverse Effects of Industry Influence." *J Am Med Assoc* 299(15) (Apr 16, 2008): 1833–5.

11. Taylor, P. "Health Care, Under the Influence." *Globe and Mail,* Toronto, ON: Apr 26, 2008.

Chapter 8. Children's Learning and Behavioral Disorders

1. "NTP Toxicology and Carcinogenesis Studies of Methylphenidate Hydrochloride" (CAS No. 298–59–9) in "F344/N Rats and B6C3F1 Mice (Feed Studies)." *Natl Toxicol Prog Tech Rep Ser* 439 (Jul 1995): 1–299.

2. Kaufman, W. *The Common Form of Joint Dysfunction: Its Incidence and Treatment.* Brattleboro, VT: E. L. Hildreth & Company, 1949.

3. Hoffer, A. *Healing Children's Attention and Behavior Disorders: Complementary Nutritional and Psychological Treatments.* Toronto, ON: CCNM Press, 2004.

4. Ibid.

5. Hoffer, A., A. W. Saul. *Orthomolecular Medicine for Everyone: Megavitamin Therapeutics for Families and Physicians.* Laguna Beach, CA: Basic Health Publications, 2008.

6. Riordan, H. D. *Medical Mavericks: Volume Three.* Wichita, KS: Bio-Communications Press, 2005

7. Saul, A. W. "The Pioneering Work of Ruth Flinn Harrell: Champion of Children." *J Orthomolecular Med* 19(1) (2004): 21–26.

8. Harrell, R. F., R. H. Capp, D. R. Davis, et al. "Can Nutritional Supplements Help Mentally Retarded Children? An Exploratory Study." *P Natl Acad Sci USA* 78 (1981): 574–578.

9. Saul. "The Pioneering Work of Ruth Flinn Harrell" *J Orthomolecular Med* 19(1): 21–26.

10. Hoffer, A., H. D. Foster. *Feel Better, Live Longer With Niacin.* Toronto, ON: CCNM Press, 2007.

11. Ieraci, A., D. G. Herrera. "Nicotinamide Protects Against Ethanol-induced Apoptolic Neurodegeneration in the Developing Mouse Brain." *PloS Med* 3(4) (Apr 2006): e101.

12. Gesch, C. B. "Food for Court: Diet and Crime." *Magistrate* 61(5) (2005): 137–139.

13. Ibid.

14. Gesch, C. B., S. M. Hammond, S. E. Hampson, et al. "Influence of Supplementary Vitamins, Minerals and Essential Fatty Acids on the Antisocial Behavior of Young Adult Prisoners. Randomized, Placebo-controlled Trial." *Brit J Psychiat* 181 (2002): 22–28.

15. Challem, J. "Mean Streets or Mean Minerals?" *The Nutrition Report 2001*. http://www.thenutritionreporter.com/Nutrition_and_Crime.html

Chapter 9. Mental Illness

1. National Park Service, USA. "Aviation: From Sand Dunes to Sonic Booms: Wright Brothers," http://www.nps.gov/nr/travel/aviation/wrightbrothers.htm

2. Hoffer, A. *Healing Schizophrenia: Complementary Vitamin and Drug Treatments.* Toronto, ON: CCNM Press, 2004.

3. Miller, C. L., J. R. Dulay. "The High-affinity Niacin Receptor HM74A Is Decreased in the Anterior Cingulate Cortex of Individuals With Schizophrenia." *Brain Res Bull* 77(1) (Sep 5, 2008): 33–41.

4. Hawkins, R., L. Pauling. *Orthomolecular Psychiatry.* San Francisco, CA: WH Freeman, 1973.

5. Miller, Dulay. "The High-affinity Niacin Receptor HM74A" *Brain Res Bull* 77(1): 33–41.

6. Hoffer, A., H. D. Foster. *Feel Better, Live Longer With Vitamin B₃: Nutrient Deficiency and Dependency.* Toronto, ON: CCNM Press, 2007.

7. Miller, C. L., P. Murakami, I. Ruczinski, et al. "Two Complex Genotypes Relevant to the Kynurenine Pathway and Melanotropin Function Show Association With Schizophrenia and Bipolar Disorder." *Schizophr Res* 113(2–3) (Sep 2009): 259–67.

8. Miller, Dulay. "The High-affinity Niacin Receptor HM74A" *Brain Res Bull* 77(1): 33–41.

9. Lorenzen, A., C. Stannek, H. Lang, et al. "Characterization of a G protein-coupled Receptor for Nicotinic Acid." *Mol Pharmacol* 2001 Feb;59(2):349–57.

10. Pike, N. B., A. Wise. "Identification of a Nicotinic Acid Receptor: Is This the Molecular Target for the Oldest Lipid-lowering Drug?" *Curr Opin Investig Drugs* 5(3) (Mar 2004): 271–5.

11. el-Zoghby, S. M., A. K. el-Shafei, G. A. Abdel-Tawab, et al. "Studies on the Effect of Reserpine Therapy on the Functional Capacity of the Tryptophan-niacin Pathway in Smoker and Non-smoker Males." *Biochem Pharmacol* 19(5) (May 1970): 1661–7.

12. Liu, C. M., S. S. Chang, S. C. Liao, et al. "Absent Response to Niacin Skin Patch

Is Specific to Schizophrenia and Independent of Smoking." *Psychiat Res* 152(2–3) (Aug 30, 2007): 181–7.

13. Hoffer, A., H. D. Foster. "Why Schizophrenics Smoke but Have a Lower Incidence of Lung Cancer: Implications for the Treatment of Both Disorders." *J Orthomolecular Med* 15 3rd Q 2000. Full text at: http://orthomolecular.org/library/jom/2000/pdf/2000-v15n03-p141.pdf

14. Prousky, J. E. "Vitamin B$_3$ for Nicotine Addiction." *J Orthomolecular Med* 19 1st Q 2004. 56. Full text at: http://www.orthomolecular.org/library/jom/2004/pdf/2004-v19n01-p056.pdf

15. Agnew, N., A. Hoffer: "Nicotinic Acid Modified Lysergic Acid Diethylamide Psychosis." *J Ment Sci* 101 (1955): 12–27.

16. Lewis, N. D., Z. A. Piotrowski. "Clinical Diagnosis of Manic-depressive Psychosis." *P Am Psychopathol Assoc* (1952–1954): 25–8.

17. Weiser, M., A. Reichenberg, J. Rabinowitz, et al. "Association Between Nonpsychotic Psychiatric Diagnoses in Adolescent Males and Subsequent Onset of Schizophrenia." *Arch Gen Psychiat* 58(10) (Oct 2001): 959–64.

18. Redelmeier, D. A., D. Thiruchelvam, N. Daneman. "Delirium After elective Surgery Among Elderly Patients Taking Statins." *Can Med Assoc J* 179(7) (Sep 23, 2008): 645–52.

19. Marcantonio, E. R. "Statins and Postoperative Delirium." *Can Med Assoc J* 179(7) (Sep 23, 2008): 627–8.

Chapter 10. Cardiovascular Disease

1. Wachter, K. "National Heart, Lung, and Blood Institute Halts Niacin Study Early; No Added Reduction in CV Events." *Internal Medicine News Digital Network* May 26, 2011. http://www.internalmedicinenews.com/news/cardiovascular-disease/single-article/nhlbi-halts-niacin-study-early-no-added-reduction-in-cv-events/2ad2602b09.html

2. Altschul, R., I. H. Herman. "Influence of Oxygen Inhalation on Cholesterol Metabolism." *Arch Biochem Biophys* 1954 51(1) (Jul): 308–9.

3. Altschul, R., A. Hoffer, J. D. Stephen. "Influence of Nicotinic Acid on Serum Cholesterol in Man." *Arch Biochem Biophys* 54 (1955): 558–559.

4. Simonson, E., A. Keys. "Research in Russia on Vitamins and Atherosclerosis." *Circulation* (Nov 24, 1961): 1239–48.

5. Grundy, Grundy, Mok, et al. "Influence of Nicotinic Acid" *J Lipid Res* 1: 24–36.

6. Wilson, B. *The Vitamin B$_3$ Therapy: A Second Communication to A. A.'s Physicians* (1968).

7. Boyle, E. "Niacin and the Heart." Paper Delivered at Int. Conf. Alcoholics Anony-

mous Physicians, New York, 1967 (excerpted in *A Second Communication to A. A.'s Physicians,* Bedford Hills, NY: 1968).

8. National Institutes of Health. NIH Consensus Development Conference Statement. "Lowering Blood Cholesterol to Prevent Heart Disease." 5(7) December 10–12, 1984. Final Panel Statement.

9. National Institutes of Health. NIH Consensus Development Program. http://consensus.nih.gov/1984/1984Cholesterol047html.htm

10. Saul, A. W. "Orthomolecular Medicine on the Internet." *J Orthomolecular Med,* 20(2) (2005): 70–74.

11. Illingworth, D. R., B. E. Phillipson, J. H. Rapp, et al. "Colestipol Plus Nicotinic Acid in Treatment of Heterozygous Familial Hypercholesterolaemia." *Lancet.* 1(8215) (Feb 7, 1981): 296–8.

12. Kane, J. P., M. J. Malloy, P. Tun, et al. "Normalization of Low-density-lipoprotein Levels in Heterozygous Familial Hypercholesterolemia With a Combined Drug Regimen." *New Engl J Med* 304(5) (Jan 29, 1981): 251–8.

13. Cheraskin, E., W. M. Ringsdorf, Jr. "The Biologic Parabola: A Look at Serum Cholesterol." *J Amer Med Assoc* 247(3) (Jan 15, 1982): 302.

14. Ueshima, H., M. Iida, Y. Komachi. "Is It Desirable to Reduce Total Serum Cholesterol Level as Low as Possible?" *Prev Med* 8(1) (Jan 1979): 104–5.

15. Hoffer, A., M. J. Callbeck. "The Hypocholesterolemic Effect of Nicotinic Acid and Its Relationship to the Autonomic Nervous System." *J Ment Sci* 103 (1957): 810–820.

16. Hoffer, A., P. O. O'Reilly, M. J. Callbeck. "Specificity of the Hypocholesterolemic Activity of Nicotinic Acid." *Dis Nerv Syst* 20 (1959): 286–288.

17. O'Reilly, P. O., M. J. Callbeck, A. Hoffer. "Sustained-Release Nicotinic Acid (Nicospan). Effect on (1) Cholesterol Levels and (2) Leukocytes." *Can Med Assoc J* 80: 359–362, 1959.

18. El-Enein, A. M. A., Y. S. Hafez, H. Salem, et al. "The Role of Nicotinic Acid and Inositol Hexanicotinate as Anti-cholesterolemic and Antilipemic Agents." *Nutrition Rep Int* 28 (1983): 899–911.

19. Mahadoo, J., L. B. Jaques, C. J. Wright. "Lipid metabolism: the histamine-glycosaminoglycan-histaminase connection." *Med Hypotheses* 7(8) (Aug 1981): 1029–38.

20. Szatmari, A., A. Hoffer, R. Schneider. "The Effect of Adrenochrome and Niacin on the Electroencephalogram of Epileptics." *Am J Psychiatry* 111(8) (Feb 1955): 603–16.

21. Hoffer, A., H. Osmond. "A Perceptual Hypothesis of Schizophrenia." *Psychiatry Dig* 28(3) (Mar 1967): 47–53.

22. Goldsborough, C. E. "Nicotinic Acid in the Treatment of Ischaemic Heart Disease." *Lancet* 2 (1960): 675–677.

23. Inkeles, S., D. Eisenberg. "Hyperlipidemia and Coronary Atherosclerosis: A Review." *Medicine (Baltimore)* (60(2) (Mar 1981): 110–23.

24. Maynard, K. I. "Natural Neuroprotectants After Stroke." *Sci Med* 8(5) (Jun 28, 2008): 258–267.

25. Mason, M. "An Old Cholesterol Remedy Is New Again." *New York Times* January 23, 2007. http://www.nytimes.com/2007/01/23/health/23consume.html?_r=1&oref=slogin

26. Adams, M. "Vitamin B$_3$ Beats Big Pharma's Zetia Cholesterol Drug." NaturalNews.com, March 30, 2010, http://www.naturalnews.com/028473_Zetia_Vitamin_B3.html

Chapter 11. Other Clinical Conditions That Respond to Niacin

1. Canner, P. L., K. G. Berge, N. K. Wenger, et al. "Fifteen Year Mortality in Coronary Drug Project Patients: Long-term Benefit With Niacin." *J Am Coll Cardiol* 8(6) (Dec 1986): 1245–55.

2. Ames, B. N., J. Elson-Schwab, E. A. Silver. "High-dose Vitamin Therapy Stimulates Variant Enzymes With Decreased Coenzyme-binding Affinity (Increased K(m)): Relevence to Genetic Disease and Polymorphism." *Am J Clin Nutr* 75 (2002): 616–658.

3. Ames, B. N. "Increasing Longevity By Tuning Up Metabolism." *Eur Mol Org* 6 (2005): S20-S24.

4. Gutierrez, H. "Micronutrient Deficiency Responsible for Cancer and other Diseases, Proclaims Scientist." NaturaNews.com November 4, 2008 http://www.naturalnews.com/024703_cancer_deficiency_health.html

5. Pauling, L. *How to Live Longer and Feel Better.* Corvallis, OR: Oregon State University Press, 2006.

6. Wysong, P. "High HDL Cholesterol May Protect Against Dementia." *Medical Post* Toronto, ON: August 10, 2004.

7. Westphal, C. H., M. A. Dipp, L. Guarente. "A Therapeutic Role for Sirtuins in Diseases of Aging?" *Trends Biochem Sci* 32(12) (December 1, 2007): 555–560.

8. Kaneko, S., J. Wang, M. Kaneko, et al. "Protecting Axonal Degeneration by Increasing Nicotinamide Adenine Dinucleotide Levels in Experimental Autoimmune Encephalomyelitis Models." *J Neurosci* 26(38) (Sep 20, 2006): 9794–804.

9. Sasaki, Y., A. Toshiyuki, J. Milbrandt. "Stimulation of Nicotinamide Adenine Dinucleotide Biosynthetic Pathways Delays Axonal Degeneration after Axotomy." *J Neurosci* 26(33) (August 16, 2006): 8484–8491.

10. Yang, H., T. Yang, J. A. Baur, et al. "Nutrient-sensitive Mitochondrial NAD+ Levels Dictate Cell Survival." *Cell* 130(6) (Sep 21, 2007): 1095–107.

11. Silverman, D. H. S., C. J. Dy, S. A. Castellon, et al. "Altered Frontocortical, Cerebellar, and Basal Ganglia Activity in Adjuvant-treated Breast Cancer Survivors 5–10 Years After Chemotherapy." *Breast Cancer Res Tr* 103(3) (Jul 2007): 303–11. Epub 2006 Sep 29.

12. Silverman, D. H. S., S. A. Castellon, P. A. Ganz. "Cognitive Dysfunction Associated With Chemotherapy for Breast Cancer." *Future Neurol* 2(3) (May 2007): 271–277.

13. Hoffer, A., A. W. Saul. *Orthomolecular Medicine for Everyone: Megavitamin Therapeutics for Families and Physicians*. Laguna Beach, CA: Basic Health Publications, 2008.

14. Hoffer, A., A. W. Saul. *The Vitamin Cure for Alcoholism*. Laguna Beach, CA: Basic Health Publications, 2008.

15. Junqueira-Franco, M. V. M., L. E. Troncon, P. G. Chiarello, et al. "Intestinal Permeability and Oxidative Stress in Patients with Alcoholic Pellagra." *Clin Nutr* 25 (2006): 977–983.

16. CBC News. "Lower-status Monkeys More Likely to Opt for Cocaine Over Food: Study." http://www.cbc.ca/news/technology/story/2008/04/07/monkeys-cocaine.html

17. ScienceDaily. "Subordinate Monkeys More Likely To Choose Cocaine Over Food." *ScienceDaily* (Apr 7, 2008). http://www.sciencedaily.com/releases/2008/04/080406153354.htm

18. Williams, R. J., M. K. Roach. "Impaired and Inadequate Glucose Metabolism in the Brain as an Underlying Cause of Alcoholism—An Hypothesis." *P Natl Acad Sci USA* 56(2) (Aug 1966): 566–571. http://www.pubmedcentral.gov/articlerender.fcgi?artid=224410

19. Foster H. D. *What Really Causes Alzheimer's Disease*. Victoria, BC: Trafford Publishing, 2004. http://www.hdfoster.com/publications

20. Morris, M. C., D. A. Evans, P. A. Bienias, et al. "Dietary Niacin and the Risk of Incident Alzheimer's Disease and of Cognitive Decline." *J Neurol Psychiatry* 75 (2004): 1093–1099.

21. Green, K. N., J. S. Steffan, H. Martinez-Coria, et al. "Nicotinamide Restores Cognition in Alzheimer's' Disease Transgenic Mice via a Mechanism Involving Soirtuin Inhibition and Selective Reduction of Thr231-Phosphotau." *J Neurosci* 45 (2008): 11500 to11510.

22. Foster. *What Really Causes Alzheimer's Disease*. http://www.hdfoster.com/publications

23. Evans, D. A., J. L. Bienias, et al. "Dietary Niacin and the Risk of Incident Alzheimer's Disease and of Cognitive Decline." *Neurol Neurosurg Psychiat* 75 (2004):1093–1099.

24. Zandi, P. P., J. C. Anthony, A. S. Khachaturian, et al. "Reduced Risk of Alzheimer Disease in Users of Antioxidant Vitamin Supplements: The Cache County Study." *Arch Neurol* 61 (2004): 82–88.

25. Thiel, R. J. "Orthomolecular Therapy and Down Syndrome: Rationale and Clinical Results." Presentation at the 8th Annual Scientific Program of the Orthomolec-

ular Health-Medicine Society, San Francisco, CA: March 1, 2002. http://www.health research.com/orthods.htm

26. Pauling, L. *How to Live Longer and Feel Better*. Corvallis, OR: Oregon State University Press, 2006. Used with permission of the Linus Pauling Institute, Oregon Sate University.

27. MacLeod, K. *Down Syndrome and Vitamin Therapy*. Ottowa, ON: Kemanso Publishing, 2003.

28. Li, J., M. Zhu, A. B. Manning-Bog, et al. "Dopamine and L-dopa Disaggregate Amyloid Fibrils: Implications for Parkinson's and Alzheimer's Disease." *FASEB J* 18(9) (Jun 2004): 962–4.

29. Religa, D., H. Laudon, M. Styczynska, et al. "Amyloid ß Pathology in Alzheimer's Disease and Schizophrenia." Am J Psychiat 160 (May 2003): 867–872.

30. Purohit, D. P., D. P. Perl, V. Haroutunian, et al. "Alzheimer Disease and Related Neurodegenerative Diseases in Elderly Patients With Schizophrenia: A Postmortem Neuropathologic Study of 100 Cases." *Arch Gen Psychiat* 55 (1998): 205–211.

31. Prousky, J., A. Hoffer. *Anxiety: Orthomolecular Diagnosis and Treatment*. Toronto, ON: CCNM Press, 2006.

32. Eighth International Symposium on ADP-Ribosylation. "Niacin Nutrition, ADP-Ribosylation and Cancer." Fort Worth, Texas, June 1987.

33. Hostetler, D. "Jacobsons Put Broad Strokes in the Niacin/Cancer Picture." *The D.O.,* 28 (Aug 1987): 103–104.

34. Hoffer, A. "The Psychophysiology of Cancer." *J Asthma Res* 8 (1970): 61–76.

35. McGinnis, W. R., T. Audhya, W. J. Walsh, et al. "Discerning the Mauve Factor, Alternative Therapies in Health and Disease, Part 1." *Alt Ther* 14(2) (Mar/Apr 2008):40–51. "Part 2" 14(3) (Jun 2008): 56–63.

36. Hoffer, A., H. D. Foster, "Schizophrenia and Cancer: The Adrenochrome Balanced Morphism." *Med Hypotheses* 62 (2004): 415–419.

37. Bartleman, A., R. Jacobs, J. B. Kirkland. "Niacin Supplementation Decreases the Incidence of Alklation-induced Nonlymphocytic Leukemia in Long-Evans Rats." *Nutr Cancer* 60 (2008): 251–258.

38. Jacobsen, E. L. "Niacin Deficiency and Cancer in Women." *J Am Coll Nutr* 12 (1993): 412–416.

39. Moalem, S. *Survival of the Sickest. A Medical Maverick Discovers Why We Need Disease*. New York, NY: HarperCollins Publishers, 2007.

40. Bartleman, Jacobs, Kirkland. "Niacin Supplementation . . ." *Nutr Cancer* 60: 251–258.

41. Boyonoski, A. C., J. C. Spronck, R. M. Jacobs, et al. "Pharmacological Intakes of Niacin Increase Bone Marrow Poly(ADP-ribose) and the Latency of Ethylnitrosourea-induced Carcinogenesis in Rats." *J Nutr* 132(1) (Jan 2002): 115–20.

42. Boyonoski, A. C., J. C. Spronck, L. M. Gallacher, et al. "Niacin Deficiency Decreases Bone Marrow Poly(ADP-ribose) and the Latency of Ethylnitrosourea-induced Carcinogenesis in Rats." *J Nutr* 132(1) (Jan 2002): 108–14.

43. Boyonoski, A. C., L. M. Gallacher, M. M. ApSimon, et al. "Niacin Deficiency in Rats Increases the Severity of Ethylnitrosourea-induced Anemia and Leukopenia." *J Nutr* 130(5) (May 2000): 1102–7.

44. Sivapirabu, G., E. Yiasemides, G. M. Halliday, et al. "Topical Nicotinamide Modulates Cellular Energy Metabolism and Provides Broad-spectrum Protection Against Ultraviolet Radiation-induced Immunosuppression in Humans." *Br J Dermatol* 161(6) (Dec 2009): 1357–64.

45. Canadian Cancer Society. "More Canadian Children Surviving Cancer—Many Experience Future Health Issues; More Research Needed: Canadian Cancer Statistics. April 9, 2008.

46. Eighth International Symposium on ADP-Ribosylation. "Niacin Nutrition . . .", June 1987.

47. Kuzniarz, M., P. Mitchell, R. G. Cumming, et al. "Use of Vitamin Supplements and Cataract: the Blue Mountains Eye Study." *Am J Ophthalmol* 132(1) (2001): 19–26.

48. Chiu, C. J. "Nutritional Antioxidants and Age-related Cataract and Maculopathy." *Exp Eye Res* 84(2) (Feb 2007): 229–45.

49. Rabbani, G. H., T. Butler, P. K. Bardhan, et al. "Reduction of Fluid-loss in Cholera by Nicotinic Acid: A Randomised Controlled Trial." *Lancet* 2(8365–66) (Dec 24–31, 1983): 1439–1442.

50. Briend, A., S. K. Nath, M. Heyman, et al. "Comparative Effects of Nicotinic Acid and Nicotinamide on Cholera Toxin-induced Secretion in Rabbit Ileum." *J Diarrhoeal Dis Res* 11(2) (Jun 1993): 97–100.

51. Petersdorf, R. G., Adams, Braunwald, et al. *Harrison's Principles of Internal Medicine*, 10th ed., New York, NY: McGraw Hill, 1983.

52. Maupin, C. "Dr. Les Simpson—Rethinking the Pathogenesis of CFIDS." *The CFS Report*. http://www.cfidsreport.com/Articles/researchers/lessimpson.htm

53. Simpson, L. O. "Altered Blood Rheology in the Pathogenesis of Diabetic and Other Neuropathies." *Muscle Nerve* 11(7) (Jul 1988): 725–44.

54. Simpson, L. O." Blood Pressure and Blood Viscosity." *NZ Med J* 101(853) (Sep 14, 1988): 581.

55. Oakley, A., J. Wallace. "Hartnup Disease Presenting in an Adult." *Clin Exp Dermatol* 19(5) (Sep 1994): 407–8.

56. Cachin, M., J. L. Beaumont. [Treatment of Migraine by Nicotinic Acid]. *Sem Hop* 27(24) Mar 30, 1951): 977–9.

57. Velling, D. A., D. W. Dodick, J. J. Muir. "Sustained-release Niacin for Prevention of Migraine Headache." *Mayo Clin Proc* 78(6) (Jun 2003): 770–1.

58. Prousky, J., D. Seely. "The Treatment of Migraines and Tension-type Headaches With Intravenous and Oral Niacin (Nicotinic Acid): Systematic Review of the Literature." *Nutr J* 4:3 (2005).

59. Kaneko, S., J. Wang, M. Kaneko, et al. "Protecting Axonal Degeneration by Increasing Nicotinamide Adenine Dinucleotide Levels in Experimental Autoimmune Encephalomyelitis Models." *J Neurosci.* 26(38) (Sep 20, 2006): 9794–804. http://www.ncbi.nlm.nih.gov/entrez/query.fcgi?CMD=search&DB=pubmed

60. Rauscher, M. "Vitamin B3 May Be Useful Against MS: Animal Study." Reuters Health. http://dukeandthedoctor.com/2010/01/vitamin-b3-may-be-useful-against-ms-animal-study/

61. Mount, H. T. "Multiple Sclerosis and other Demyelinating Diseases." *Can Med Assoc J* 108(11) (Jun 2, 1973): 1356–1358.

62. Klenner, F. R. "Response of Peripheral and Central Nerve Pathology to Mega-Doses of the Vitamin B-Complex and Other Metabolites." *J Appl Nutr* 1973, http://www.tldp.com/issue/11_00/klenner.htm

63. Klenner, F. R. "Clinical Guide to the Use of Vitamin C." http://www.seanet .com/~alexs/ascorbate/198x/smith-lh-clinical_guide_1988.htm

64. Klenner, F. R. "Treating Multiple Sclerosis Nutritionally." *Cancer Control J* 2(3): 16–20.

65. "Peter's Promise" http://www.orthomolecular.com (accessed Jan 2011).

66. Wahlberg, G., L. A. Carlson, J. Wasserman, et al. "Protective Effect of Nicotinamide Against Nephropathy in Diabetic Rats." *Diabetes Res* 2 (1985): 307–312.

67. Condorelli, L. "Nicotinic Acid in the Therapy of the Cardiovascular Apparatus." In: R. Altschul, ed. *Niacin in Vascular Disorders and Hyperlipemia* Springfield, IL: CC Thomas, 1964.

68. Wald, G., B. Jackson. "Activity and Nutritional Deprivation." *P Nat Acad Sci USA,* 30(9) (Sep 15, 1944): 255–263.

69. Kaufman, W. *The Common Form of Joint Dysfunction: Its Incidence and Treatment.* Brattleboro, VT: E. L. Hildreth & Company, 1949.

70. Hoffer, A., H. D. Foster. *Feel Better, Live Longer With Vitamin B3: Nutrient Deficiency and Dependency.* Toronto, ON: CCNM Press, 2007.

71. Foster, H. D. and A. Hoffer. "The Two Faces of L-DOPA: Benefits and Adverse Side Effects in the Treatment of Encephalitis Lethargica, Parkinson's Disease, Multiple Sclerosis and Amyotrophic Lateral Sclerosis." *Med Hypotheses* 62(2) (February 2004): 177–181.

72. Hoffer, Foster. *Feel Better, Live Longer With Vitamin B3.*

73. Foster, H. D., A. Hoffer. "Hyperoxidation of the Two Catecholamines, Dopamine and Adrenaline: Implications for the Etiologies and Treatment of Encephalitis Lethargica, Parkinson's Disease, Multiple Sclerosis, Amyotrophic Lateral Sclerosis, and Schizophrenia." In: *Oxidative Stress and Neurodegenerative Disorders*, Amsterdam: Elsevier, 2007, Ch 16, 369–382.

74. Evans, E. L., P. J. Matts. Skin Care Composition Containing Glycerin and a Vitamin B_3 Compound That Increase and Repair Skin Barrier Function. Eur. Pat. Appl. (2004), EP 1459736; A1 20040922. Patent written in English.

75. Jacobson, E. L. et al. "A Topical Lipophilic Niacin Derivative Increases NAD, Epidermal Differentiation and Barrier Function in Photodamaged Skin." *Exp Dermatol* 16(6) (2007): 490–499.

76. Moro, O. Antiaging Topical Formulations Containing Niacin and Ubiquinones. Jpn. Kokai Tokkyo Koho (2005) JP 2005298370; A 20051027. Patent written in Japanese.

77. Sore, G., I. Hansenne. Peeling Composition Containing Vitamin B_3 and Vitamin C. Fr. Demande (2005), FR 2861595; A1 20050506. Patent written in French.

78. Tanno, O. "The New Efficacy of Niacinamide in the Skin and the Application to the Skin Care Products of Cosmetics." *Fragrance J* 32(2) (2004): 35–39.

79. Yates, P. R., R. L. Charles-Newsham. Skin Lightening Compositions Comprising Vitamins and Flavonoids. PCT Int. Appl. (2005), WO 2005094770; A1 20051013.

80. Hoffer, Saul. *Orthomolecular Medicine for Everyone.*

81. Tang, H., J. Y. Lu, X. Zheng, et al. "The Psoriasis Drug Monomethylfumarate Is a Potent Nicotinic Acid Receptor Agonist." *Biochem Biophys Res Commun* 375(4) (Oct 31, 2008): 562–5.

82. Hoffer A, M. Walker. *Putting It All Together: The New Orthomolecular Nutrition.* New Canaan, CT: Keats Publishing Inc., 1996. Also: McGraw-Hill; 1998.

83. Wallace, A.E., W. B. Weeks. "Thiamine Treatment of Chronic Hepatitis B Infection." *Am J Gastroenterol* 96(3) (2001): 864–868.

84. Shoji, S. et al. "Thiamine Disulfide as a Potent Inhibitor of Human Immunodeficiency Virus (Type-1) Production. Biochemical and Biophysical Research Communications." 205(1) (1994): 967–75.

85. Murray, M. F. "Niacin as a Potential AIDS Preventive Factor." *Med Hypotheses* 53(5) (1999): 375–379.

86. Tang, A. M., N. M. Graham, A. J. Kirby, et al. "Dietary Micronutrient Intake and Risk of Progression to Acquired Immunodeficiency Syndrome (AIDS) in Human Immunodeficiency Virus Type 1 (HIV-1)-Infected Homosexual Men." *Am J Epidemiol* 138(11) (Dec 1, 1993): 937–51.

87. Fawzi, W. W., G. I. Msamanga, D. Spiegelman, et al. "A Randomized Trial of

Multivitamin Supplements and HIV Disease Progression and Mortality." *New Engl J Med* 351(1) (Jul 1, 2004): 23–32.

88. Foster, H. D. What Really Causes AIDS. Victoria: Trafford Publishing, 2002

89. Foster, H. D. "Treating AIDS with Nutrition." Doctor Yourself Newsletter, 4(12) (May 20, 2004). http://www.doctoryourself.com/news/v4n12.txt

90. Bradfield, M., H. D. Foster." The Successful Orthomolecular Treatment of AIDS: Accumulating Evidence from Africa." *J Orthomolecular Med* 21(4) (2006). http://www.orthomolecular.org/library/jom/2006/pdf/2006-v21n04-p193.pdf

Appendix. The Introduction of Niacin as the First Successful Treatment for Cholesterol Control

1. Parsons, W. B. Jr, R. W. P. Achor, K. G. Berge, et al. "Changes in Concentration of Blood Lipids Following Prolonged Administration of Large Doses of Nicotinic Acid to Persons With Hypercholesterolemia: Preliminary Observations." *P Staff Meet Mayo Clinic,* 31 (1956): 377–390.

2. Altschul, R., A. Hoffer, J. D. Stephen. "Influence of Nicotinic Acid on Serum Cholesterol in Man." *Arch Biochem Biophys* 54 (1955): 558–559.

3. Altschul, R. *Niacin in Vascular Disorders and Hyperlipidemia.* Springfield, IL: Charles C. Thomas, 1964.

4. Altschul, Hoffer, Stephen. "Influence of Nicotinic acid . . ." *Arch Biochem Biophys* 1955: 558–559.

5. Parsons, W. B. Jr. *Cholesterol Control Without Diet! The Niacin Solution.* Scottsdale, AZ: Lilac Press, 1998.

6. The Coronary Drug Project Research Group. "Clofibrate and Niacin in Coronary Heart Disease." *J Am Med Assoc* 231 (1975): 360–381.

7. Canner, P. L., K. G. Berge, N. K. Wenger, et al., for the Coronary Drug Project Research Group. "Fifteen Year Mortality in Coronary Drug Project Patients: Long-term Benefit With Niacin." *J Am Coll Cardiol* 8 (1986): 1245–1255.

For Further Reading

American Society for Nutrition. "Symposium: Nutrients and Epigenetic Regulation of Gene Expression." *J Nutr* 139(12) (Dec 2009): 2397–240.

Angell, M. "Is Academic Medicine for Sale?" *N Engl J Med* 342(20) (May 18, 2000): 1516–8.

Benavente, C. A., M. K. Jacobson, E. L. Jacobson. "NAD in Skin: Therapeutic Approaches for Niacin." *Curr Pharm Des* 15(1) (Jan 2009): 29–38.

Benavente, C. A., E. L. Jacobson. "Niacin Restriction Upregulates NADPH Oxidase and Reactive Oxygen Species (ROS) in Human Keratinocytes." *Free Radic Biol Med* 44 (Feb 2008): 527–37.

Berge, K. G., P. L. Canner. "Coronary Drug Project: Experience with Niacin. Coronary Drug Project Research Group." *Eur J Clin Pharmacol* 40 Suppl 1 (1991): S49–51.

Berger, M. M. "Nutrients as Antioxidants—Effect of Antioxidative Trace Elements and Vitamins on Outcome of Critically Ill Burns and Trauma Patients." *Aktuelle Ernaehrungsmedizin* 28(6) (2003): 376–379.

Birkmayer, J. G., C. Vrecko, D. Volc, et al. "Nicotinamide Adenine Dinucleotide (NADH)—A New Therapeutic Approach to Parkinson's Disease. Comparison of Oral and Parenteral Application." *Acta Neurol Scand Suppl* 146 (1993): 32–35.

Boyle, E. "Communication to AA by Bill W." In: *The Vitamin B3 Therapy.* 1967.

Carey, J. "FDA Rejects Merck's Cordaptive." *BusinessWeek.* (April 29, 2008): 11–13.

Challem, J. *Nutrition Reporter* 19 (2008)

Clarkes, R. "Niacin for Nicotine?" *Lancet* 1(8174) (Apr 26 1980): 936.

Cleave, T. L., G. D. Campbell, N. S. Painter. *Diabetes, Coronary Thrombosis and the Saccharine Disease.* 2nd. ed. Bristol, ENG: John Wright and Sons, 1969.

DeAngelis, C. D., P. B. Fontanarosa. "Impugning the Integrity of Medical Science: The Adverse Effects of Industry Influence." *J Am Med Assoc* 299(15) (2008): 1833–1835.

El Enein, A., A. M. Hafez, Y.S. Salem, et al. "The Role of Nicotinic Acid and Inositol Hexanicotinate as Anticholesterolemic and Antilipemic Agents." *Nutr Rep Int* 281 (1983): 899–911.

Foster, H. D. "New Strategies For Reversing Vital Pandemics: The Role of Nutrition." *P Int Forum Public Health Shanghai* (2007): 19–23.

Galadari, E., S. Hadi, K. Sabarinathan. "Hartnup Disease." *Int J Dermatol.* 32(12) (Dec 1993): 904.

Graveline, D. "Transient Global Amnesia. A Side Effect of 'Statins' Treatment." *Townsend Letter for Doctors and Patients* 253/254 (Aug/Sept 2004): 85–89.

Hill, K. P., J. S. Ross, D. S. Egilman, et al. "The ADVANTAGE Seeding Trial: A Review of Internal Documents." *Ann Intern Med* 149(4) (Aug 2008): 251–258.

Hoffer, A. *Adventures in Psychiatry.* Toronto, ON: Kos Press, 2005.

Hoffer, A. *Dr. Hoffer's ABC of Natural Nutrition for Children.* Kingston, ON: Quarry Press, 1999. 45.

Hoffer, A. "Epidermolysis Bullosa: A Zinc Dependent Condition?" *J Orthomolecular Med* 7 (1992): 245–246.

Hoffer, A. *Healing Cancer.* Toronto, ON: CCNM Press, 2004.

Hoffer, A. *Hoffer's Laws of Natural Nutrition: A Guide to Eating Well for Pure Health.* Kingston, ON: Quarry Press, 1996.

Hoffer, A. "Hong Kong Veterans Study." *J Orthomolecular Psychiat* 3 (1974): 34–36.

Hoffer, A. "Mechanism of Action of Nicotinic Acid and Nicotinamide in the Treatment of Schizophrenia." In: *Orthomolecular Psychiatry,* R. Hawkins, L. Pauling, eds. San Francisco, CA WH Freeman, 1973.

Hoffer, A. *Niacin Therapy in Psychiatry.* Springfield, IL: CC Thomas, 1962.

Hoffer, A. *Mental Health Regained.* Toronto, ON: International Schizophrenia Foundation, 2007.

Hoffer, A. "An Orthomolecular Look at Obesity." *J Orthomolecular Med* 22(1st Q 2007): 4–7.

Hoffer, A. *Orthomolecular Treatment for Schizophrenia. A Keats Good Health Guide.* Lincolnwood, IL: Keats, 1999.

Hoffer, A. "The Psychophysiology of Cancer." *J Asthma Res* 8 (1970): 61–76.

Hoffer, A. *Treatment Manual.* Toronto, ON: International Schizophrenia Foundation, 2007.

Hoffer, A. *User's Guide to Natural Therapies for Cancer Prevention and Control.* Laguna Beach, CA: Basic Health Publications, 2004.

Hoffer, A. *Vitamin B₃ and Schizophrenia: Discovery, Recovery, Controversy.* Kingston, ON: Quarry Press, 2004.

Hoffer, A. *Vitamin B₃: Niacin and Its Amide.* http://www.doctoryourself.com/hoffer_niacin.html.

Hoffer, A., H. Osmond. *The Chemical Basis of Clinical Psychiatry.* Springfield, IL: CC Thomas, 1960.

Hoffer, A., H. Osmond. *The Hallucinogens.* Academic Press, New York, 1967.

Hoffer, A., H. Osmond. *How To Live With Schizophrenia.* New York, NY, University Books, 1966. (Also published by Johnson, London, ENG, 1966, written by Fannie Kahan; New revised ed.: Citadel Press, New York, NY, 1992. Revised: Quarry Press, Kingston, ON.

Hoffer, A., H. Osmond, M. J. Callbeck, I. Kahan. "Treatment of Schizophrenia With Nicotinic Acid and Nicotinamide." *J Clin Exper Psychopathol* 18(2) (1957): 131–158.

Hoffer, A., H. Osmond, J. Smythies. "Schizophrenia: A New Approach. II. Results of a Year's Research." *J Ment Sci* 100 (1954): 29–45.

Hoffer, A., J. Prousky. *Naturopathic Nutrition: A Guide to Nutrient-rich Food & Nutritional Supplements for Optimum Health.* Toronto, ON: CCNM Press, 2006.

Hoffer, A., A. W. Saul. *The Vitamin Cure for Alcoholism.* Laguna Beach, CA: Basic Health Publications, 2008.

Hoffer, A., M. Walker. *Putting It All Together: The New Orthomolecular Nutrition.* New Canaan, CT: Keats Publishing, 1996.

Horton, J. W. et al. "Antioxidant Vitamin Therapy Alters Burn Trauma-mediated Cardiac NF-B Activation and Cardiomyocyte Cytokine Secretion." *J Trauma: Inj Inf Crit Care,* 50(3) (2001): 397–408.

Jacobson, E. L., Jacobson, M. K. "A Biomarker for the Assessment of Niacin Nutriture as a Potential Preventive Factor in Carcinogenesis." *J Intern Med* 233(1) (Jan 1993): 59–62.

Jonas, A. J., I. J. Butler. "Circumvention of Defective Neutral Amino Acid Transport in Hartnup Disease Using Tryptophan Ethyl Ester." *J Clin Invest.* 84(1) (Jul 1989): 200–204.

Jonas, W. B., C. P. Rapoza, W. F. Blair. "The Effect of Niacinamide on Osteoarthritis: A Pilot Study." *Inflamm Res* 45 (1996): 330–4.

Kaufman, W. "Bibliography of Professional Publications." DoctorYourself.com. http://www.doctoryourself.com/biblio_kaufman.html

Kaufman, W. "Collected Papers." University of Michigan, Special Collections Library, 7th Floor, Harlan Hatcher Graduate Library, Ann Arbor, MI 48109. special.collections@umich.edu Phone: 734-764-9377

Kaufman, W. *Common Forms of Niacinamide Deficiency Disease: Aniacin Amidosis.* New Haven, CT: Yale University Press, 1943.

Kaufman, W. "Niacinamide Improves Mobility in Degenerative Joint Disease." *Am Assoc Adv Sci* Program, Philadelphia, PA: AAAS, May 24–30, 1986. Abstract.

Kaufman. W. "Niacinamide Therapy for Joint Mobility." *Conn. State Med. J* 17 (1953): 584–589.

Kaufman, W. "Vitamin Deficiency, Megadoses, and Some Supplemental History." (1992) Letter. DoctorYourself.com. http://www.doctoryourself.com/kaufman2.html

Kaufman, W. "What Took So Long to Come Out in Favor of Folic Acid?" Commentary. DoctorYourself.com. http://www.doctoryourself.com/kaufman4.html

Kirkland, J. B. "Niacin Status Impacts Chromatin Structure." *J Nutr* 139(12) (Dec 2009): 2397–2401.

Kunin, R. A. "The Action of Aspirin in Preventing the Niacin Flush and Its Relevance to the Antischizophrenic Action of Megadose Niacin." *J Orthomolecular Psychiat* 5 (1976): 89–100.

Lewis, N. D. C., Z. A. Piotrowski. "Clinical Diagnosis of Manic-depressive Psychosis." In: *Depression,* P. H. Hoch, J. Zubin, eds., New York, NY: Grune & Stratton, 1954. 25–38.

Linus Pauling Institute, Micronutrient Information Center. Oregon State University. J. Higdon 2002; Updated by V. J. Drake 2007. lpi.oregonstate.edu/infocenter/vitamins/niacin

McCarty, M. F. "Co-administration of Equimolar Doses of Betaine May Alleviate the Hepatotoxic Risk Associated With Niacin Therapy." *Med Hypotheses* 55 (2000): 189–194.

McCracken, R. D. *Niacin and Human Health Disorders.* Fort Collins, CO: Hygea Publishing Co., 1994.

McIlroy, A. "A Tip to Get That Monkey off Your Back." *Globe and Mail,* April 7, 2008.

Miller, C. L., I. C. Llenos, J. R. Dulay, et al. "Expression of the Kynurenine Pathway Enzmye Tryptophan 2.3 Dioxygenase is Increased in the Frontal Cortex of Individuals With Schizophrenia." *Neurobiol Dis* 15 (2004): 618–629.

Miller, C. L., I. C. Llenos, J. R. Dulay, et al. "Upregulation of the Initiating Step of the Kynurenine Pathway in Postmortem Anterior Cingulate Cortex from Individuals With Schizophrenia and Bipolar disorders." *Brain Res* 1073–1074 (2006): 25–37.

Morris, M. C., D. A. Evans, J. L. Bienias, et al. "Dietary Intake of Antioxidant Nutrients and the Risk of Incident Alzheimer's Disease in a Biracial Community Study." *J Am Med Assoc* 287(24) (2002): 3230–3237.

Munro, M. "Cholesterol Pill's Side Effects Worry BBC Drug Specialists." Victoria, BC: *Times-Colonist,* September 16, 2003.

Murray, M. F. *Treatment of Retrovirus Induced Derangements With Niacin Compounds.* Cambridge, MA: The Foundation for Innovative Therapies. 9 p.

Murray, M. F., M. Langan, R. R. MacGregor. "Increased Plasma Tryptophan in HIV-infected Patients Treated With Pharmacologic Doses of Nicotinamide." *Nutrition* (NY) 17(7/8) (2001): 654–656.

Parsons, W. B., Jr. "The Effect of Nicotinic Acid on the Liver. Evidence Favoring Functional Alteration of Enzymatic Reactions Without Hepatocellular Damage." In: *Niacin in Vascular Disorders and Hyperlipemia.* R Altshul, ed. Springfield, IL: CC Thomas, 1964.

Parsons, W. B., Jr., R. W. P. Achor, K. G. Berge, et al. "Changes in Concentration of Blood Lipids Following Prolonged Administration of Large Doses of Nicotinic Acid to Persons with Hypercholesterolemia: Preliminary Observations." *Proc Staff Meet Mayo Clinic*, 31 (1956): 377–390.

Picard, A. "Beating Cancer: the Good and the Bad." *Globe and Mail,* Toronto, ON: April 10, 2008.

Prousky, J., C. G. Millman, J. J. Kirkland. "Pharmacologic Use of Niacin." *J Evidence-Based Complementary Alt Med* 16(2) (March 24, 2011): 91–101.

Saul, A. "Down Syndrome: The Nutritional Treatment of Henry Turkel, M.D." DoctorYourself.com. http://www.doctoryourself.com/turkel.html

Schmidtke, K., W. Endres, A. Roscher, et al. "Hartnup Syndrome, Progressive Encephalopathy and Allo-albuminaemia. A Clinico-pathological Case Study." *Eur J Pediatr* 151(12) (Dec 1992): 899–903.

Silverman, D. H. S. "Altered Bain Function After Chemotherapy." *Neurol Rev* 14(11) (2006).

Silverman, D. H. S. "Changes in Brain Function Persist 10 Years after Chemotherapy, Imaging Study Suggests." *Oncology Times* 28(2225) (November 2006): 50.

Simpson, L. O. "Can the Role of Statins be Discussed Without Recognition of Their Effects on Blood Viscosity? Rapid Response." *BMJ* April 3, 2008.

Spies, T. D., C. D. Aring, J. Gelperin, et al. "The Mental Symptoms of Pellagra: Their Relief with Nicotinic Acid." *Am J Med Sci* 196 (1938): 461.

Spies, T. D., W. B. Bean, R. E. Stone. "The Treatment of Subclinical and Classical Pellagra: Use of Nicotinic Acid, Nicotinic Acid Amide and Sodium Nicotinate, with Special Reference to the Vasodilator Action and Effect on Mental Symptoms." *J Am Med Assoc* 111 (1938): 581.

Stroup, T. S., J. P. McEvoy, M. S. Swartz, et al. "The National Institute of Mental Health Clinical Antipsychotic Trials of Intervention Effectiveness (CATIE) project: Schizophrenia Trial Design and Protocol Development." *Schizophr Bull* 29(1) (2003): 15–31.

Taubes, G. *Good Calories, Bad Calories* New York, NY: Knopf, 2007.

Titus, K. "Scientists Link Niacin and Cancer Prevention." *The D.O.* 28 (Aug 1987): 93–97.

Taylor, P. "Bad Medicine: Health Care, Under the Influence." *Globe and Mail* April 26, 2008.

Turkel, H. "Medical amelioration of Down syndrome incorporating the orthomolecular approach." *J Orthomolecular Psych* 4 (1975):102–115.

Turkel, H. "Medical amelioration of Down syndrome incorporating the orthomolecular approach," in: *Diet Related to Killer Diseases V. Nutrition and Mental Health*. Hearing before the Select Committee on Nutrition and Human Needs of the United States Senate, Washington, DC: U.S. Government Printing Office, 1977: 291–304.

Turkel, H. *Medical treatment of Down syndrome and genetic diseases,* Southfield, MI: Ubiotica, 4th rev. ed., 1985.

Turkel, H. *New hope for the mentally retarded: Stymied by the FDA.* New York, NY: Vantage Press, 1972.

Uneri, O., U. Tural, N. Cakin Memik. "Smoking and Schizophrenia: Where is the Biological Connection." *Turk Psikiyatri Dergisi* 17 (2006): 1–10.

Wald, G., B. Jackson. "Activity and Nutritional Deprivation." *P Natl Acad Sci USA* 30(9) (Sep 15 1944): 255–263.

Wilson, B. *The Vitamin B₃ Therapy: The First Communication to A.A.'s Physicians,* Bedford Hills, NY: 1967. Private publication.

Wilson, B. *A second communication to A.A.'s physicians.* Bedford Hills, NY:/Private publication. 1968.

Wittenborn, J. R., E. S. P. Weber, M. Brown. "Niacin in the Long Term Treatment of Schizophrenia." *Arch Gen Psychiat* 28 (1973): 308–315.

Yamada, K., K. Nonaka, T. Hanafusa, et al. "Preventive and Therapeutic Effects of Large-dose Nicotinamide Injections on Diabetes Associated With Insulitis." *Diabetes* 31 (1982): 749–753.

Yang, J., J. D. Adams. "Nicotinamide and Its Pharmacological Properties for Clinical Therapy." *Drug Design Rev* 1 (2004): 43–52.

Yang, J., L. K. Klaidman, J. D. Adams. "Medicinal Chemistry of Nicotinamide in the Treatment of Ischemis and Reperfusion." *Mini-Rev Med Chem* 2 (2002): 125–134.

Yu, B., Zhao, S. "Anti-inflammatory Effect is an Important Property of Niacin on Atherosclerosis Beyond Its Lipid-altering Effects." *Med Hypotheses* 69(1) (2007): 90–94.

Zandi, P. P. "Vitamin C, E in High Dose Combination May Protect Against Alzheimer's Disease." FuturePundit: Future technological trends and their likely effects on human society, politics and evolution. January 20, 2004. http://www.futurepundit.com/archives/001899.html

Index

About the Authors

Abram Hoffer, M.D., Ph.D. (1917–2009)
Orthomolecular Medicine Hall of Fame 2006
Dr. Rogers Prize, 2007

In the documentary film, *Masks of Madness: Science of Healing*, Abram Hoffer says: "Mental illness is usually biochemical illness. Schizophrenia is niacin dependency." Plain-spoken statements such as these have ignited a revolution in psychiatry. The person who would forever change the course of medicine was born on a Saskatchewan farm and educated in a one-room schoolhouse. In 1952, just completing his residency, he demonstrated with the first double-blind, placebo-controlled studies in the history of psychiatry that vitamin B₃ could cure schizophrenia. But in a medical profession that "knows" vitamins do not cure "real" diseases, the young director of psychiatric research was a dissenter. For over half a century Dr. Hoffer would continue to dissent. Harold Foster wrote: "Fathering a new paradigm does not promote popularity. Fortunately, Dr. Hoffer is not just highly intelligent; he has consistently proven to be able to stand up for the truth, regardless of personal cost."

"If patients look up 'schizophrenia' in the old textbooks," said Dr. Hoffer, "they'll die of frustration and fear. That is why I wrote my first book, *How to Live with Schizophrenia*. Linus Pauling was sixty-five and planning to retire. He chanced to see this book on a friend's coffee table. Pauling did not go to bed the first night he read this book. He decided not to retire because of it."

Dr. Hoffer wrote over thirty books and over 600 papers. He created the

226

Journal of Orthomolecular Medicine and was its editor-in-chief for four decades. Having treated thousands of patients, he finally retired at age eighty-eight, wryly saying that "Everyone should have a career change every fifty-five years."

Linus Pauling said, "Abram Hoffer has made an important contribution to the health of human beings. . . through the study of the effects of large doses of vitamins and other nutrients."

Andrew W. Saul (b. 1955)
Citizens for Health Outstanding Health Freedom Activist Award, 1994

Andrew Saul has taught nutrition, health science, and cell biology at the college level. He is editor of the *Orthomolecular Medicine News Service* and the author of the Basic Health Publications, Inc. books *Doctor Yourself* and *Fire Your Doctor!* He wrote *Orthomolecular Medicine for Everyone* and *The Vitamin Cure for Alcoholism* with Dr. Abram Hoffer. He is coauthor of four other books: *Vitamin C: The Real Story; The Vitamin Cure for Children's Health Problems; I Have Cancer: What Should I Do?* and *Hospitals and Health*. Dr. Saul is series editor for Basic Health's *Vitamin Cure* book series. He is on the editorial board of the *Journal of Orthomolecular Medicine* and is featured in the documentary film *Food Matters*. He has twice won New York Empire State Fellowship for teaching, and has published over 100 reviews and editorials in peer-reviewed publications. His internationally famous noncommercial natural healing website is DoctorYourself.com.

Harold D. Foster, Ph.D. (1943–2009)
Orthomolecular Medicine Hall of Fame 2010

Harold Foster was deeply invested in improving the quality of life for all living things. For more than forty years, Dr. Foster worked as a geomorphologist, professor of medical geography, consultant to the United Nations and NATO in disaster planning, and avid researcher, which culminated in the formation of the Harold Foster Foundation.

A Canadian by choice, Dr. Foster was born in Tunstall, Yorkshire, England, and educated at the Hull Grammar School and University College London. While at university, he specialized in geology and geography, earning a B.Sc. in 1964 and a Ph.D. in 1968. He was a faculty member in the Department of Geography, University of Victoria, from 1967 to 2008. As a tenured professor, he authored or edited over 300 publications, the majority of which focused on reducing disaster losses or identifying the causes of chronic degenerative and infectious diseases.

His numerous books include *Disaster Planning: The Preservation of Life and Property; Health, Disease and the Environment,* and *Reducing Cancer Mortality: A Geographical Perspective.* He also wrote six books in the What Really Causes series, including those on AIDS, Alzheimer's disease, multiple sclerosis, schizophrenia, SIDS, and breast cancer. Dr. Foster made unique contributions in our understanding of health and disease as he explored the complex relationships between genetic inheritance, health and the "nutritional geographies" of the world. He also conducted many groundbreaking studies of selenium in AIDS therapy in Africa.

Dr. Foster served on the editorial board of the *Journal of Orthomolecular Medicine* for fifteen years, and on the board of directors for the International Schizophrenia Foundation for thirteen years.